The Fasting Highway

The Fasting Highway

Get into the passenger seat beside intermittent fasting advocate Graeme Currie from Australia as he takes you on a journey through the highs and lows of beating a crippling food addiction by losing 60kg (132lb) and a lifetime's worth of poor self-esteem.

As featured on intermittent fasting Stories Podcast Episode 23 with Host Gin Stephens Author of "Delay Don't Deny" and New York Times Best Seller "Fast, Feast, Repeat"

GRAEME CURRIE

THE FASTING HIGHWAY

Cover design and layout: Eled Cernik

ISBN: 978-0-6489652-0-6

I am not a doctor nor am I a trained health professional.
Any of the written content in my personal story that follows should not be considered as medical advice.
Please consult with your doctor or trained medical professional before starting any health plan. I have no affiliations with any product or health related companies.

TABLE OF CONTENTS

INTRODUCTION

Hello and thank you for getting into the passenger seat with me on this warts-and-all journey from addiction to control.

My name's Graeme and I'm just a regular working-class guy who has battled with obesity and food addiction his whole life. I wrote this book to show you what can happen when an average person like me reaches the depths of despair and makes a choice to take back control of his life.

The choice that I made in that dark hour, resulted in my discovery of intermittent fasting as an eating philosophy, which took my weight from a high of 160 kg (352 pounds) to its current level of 100kg (220 pounds) which I have been able to comfortably maintain well for nearly two years.

I chose the name The Fasting Highway for this book, because for me, intermittent fasting became a relatively fast, clearly signposted route to success and a big change from the narrow, winding lanes which attempts at controlling my eating had taken me down, frequently ending in wrong turns and dead ends.

I should tell you that my style of writing is casual. I didn't want to write a book bogged down with the science behind intermittent fasting because quite frankly, this is not my area of expertise. I don't know all of the ins and outs of the science, but I do know what goes on behind the smiling façade of someone who is morbidly obese and addicted to all the wrong foods, desperate to stop making the same mistakes.

If you've experienced similar issues, you may see yourself in some of my story and if the sharing of this story helps motivate even one other person to take control of their life and turn their health around, then I will consider it to have been a success.

CHAPTER 1

Back Story to My Life as an Obese Person

Anyone who has been obese or carried lots of weight knows what sort of burden that can be.

Writing this book has been an emotional time for me with a lot of soul searching, as it brought back to me many painful memories of how my obesity had caused so much heartache, hurt, and embarrassment that resulted in me having such a low opinion of myself. It is still amazing to me, when I put it all together, how far away from happy I became, all because of food.

We all know the names obese people cruelly get called. Over the years I have heard them all- fat, fatty, slob, freak, chubs, lard ass, beach ball, just to name just a few. We all know the deep hurt of overhearing people commenting about your weight in public. Or the street vendor overseas selling t-shirts that scream out, "Hey! You don't have to worry; we have jumbo size here."

I endured years of sniggering, laughing, and teasing by those mean kids or workmates. I was often told I was too fat for something or I was too heavy for that ride. Then there were those kids that would yell at the top of their voices, "look at that fat guy" on public transport. I was never ever picked on a team at school during lunchtime sport because I was the fat kid who couldn't run. Fat kids are always trying to make themselves invisible to just fit in. We all know obesity is a crushing burden and all I can tell you is once you are not obese and that very heavy burden is lifted, it's like freedom I have never experienced and it's liberating once you get rid of the weight.

> **I have been asked a lot why I got to be so obese. Normal people cannot understand why you just don't eat better food.**

Why can't you just stop? In my mind, sugar and fast food were the main contributors to my obesity. I want to make it clear I don't want to demonise sugar and fast food at all in this book. I truly respect people's right to eat whatever they want. I know I had a very big problem with sugar and fast food myself, I was addicted to them. There was no such thing as moderation with me. I ate as much as I could stuff into my mouth regularly and often. Unfortunately, for some us, there is no such thing as balance and moderation. I had no self-control with sugar and an insatiable appetite for fast food and carbohydrates like bread and potato chips.

I think all of us know deep down why we are obese. We are the ones stuffing ourselves all day. We just ignore those signals that our bodies give us because our desire for that hit of fast food and sugar is so ingrained in us it overrides everything.

Some people have a genuine medical issue that causes weight gain. Amazingly, I never had any medical problems relating to the excess weight I was carrying. I was never diabetic or even pre-diabetic at my heaviest weight. I just couldn't stop eating foods that made me fatter each year.

It didn't help in my teen years my parents owned a convenience store in New Zealand and I ate and drank myself stupid daily and stacked on the weight. My parents worked hard, and I would often take food from the shop and eat it in secret in the flat upstairs. The bigger I got, the more unhappy and withdrawn I got. I had few friends and never had a girlfriend in high school. I was the victim of some bad bullying at school by teachers and kids. I was that big obese kid that everyone thought it was ok to ridicule, tease and abuse every day. I got into a lot of fights – some I won, but usually I would be fighting a pack of boys who just wanted to give the fat kid a kicking.

> **After I left school, I staggered from job to job and the bullying and discrimination carried on.**

I got very ill at 19 with rheumatic fever and came close to dying in the hospital. I lost a huge amount of weight through being ill, and, when I recovered, I found a new job. People reacted so differently to me without all the weight. I became a social butterfly, met lots of girls, and partied a lot as a young person does. It was my first taste of what it was like as a normal sized person. I never got bullied, I was popular and had a lot of friends.

Eventually, though, the weight returned, and through my 20s, 30s, 40s, and 50s I just got bigger. I did not exercise or pay any attention to my diet whatsoever. I just ate whatever I wanted and had no off button. I became morbidly obese past that tipping point where I just accepted this was my lot in life. I developed chronic addictions to sugar and fast food that set the foundation for decades of gluttony and closet eating issues. I lived all my adult years nearly as a morbidly obese man and that I have a lot of regret and guilt about. I never thought I would get a second go at life so full of health and get my weight to a sustainable point of wellness.

I thought about food pretty much all day for years – where could I get my next snack, my next soft drink or meal from. I would no sooner finish one meal than I would start thinking about the next one. I was also the eternal snacker, often having multiple snacks throughout the day. These snacks were often the size of a meal in themselves.

> **I would eat breakfast most days at home, before leaving the house to drive to work. I wouldn't get ten minutes down the street before pulling into the local fast-food drive-through.**

I would order toasted sandwiches and a giant coffee to have on my commute to work. Some days I just didn't do that once on my 50-minute commute, I'd do it twice. It was ok, no one could see me I was in my car and that was my haven. I could eat as much as I liked in there with no one judging me or seeing me.

Often, for good measure, after I ate the fast food, I sometimes ate that bag of potato chips I had stashed under the seat. I was eating breakfast twice, lunch, afternoon tea, a meal on the way home, and then dinner at home with a dessert. I was really an eating machine all day. I had no off button whatsoever, and just ate whenever I could get the opportunity.

> **Once I was at the office, I would be that guy who acted like he never ate anything at the office.**

I would loudly decline the party cakes people bought into work to make it look like I was abstemious. That was because I would wait till, they went home and then eat the leftovers. True story. With my size, I don't know who I thought I was fooling that I was a moderate, mindful eater.

On my commute home, I often couldn't help myself. Knowing full well that I had a lovely dinner waiting for me at home, I would still turn into the drive-through and pick up something to have on my way home, more snacks. Those signs drew me in like a magnet. I would be determined every day not to go through them, and then, every day without fail, there I was, in the cue for my fix. I hated myself when I was in the cue waiting to order, but I just had to get that food, and it was often a relief when I took that first bite. It sure had a hold on me and my mind. Everything I did was driven by food. My shirts and jackets pants were always stained with food, and it was a dead giveaway of the eating sessions in my car.

Addicts find ways to eat a lot of food secretly, and dread being found out how much they do eat.

By hiding food, you hide how much you really do eat, a bit like hiding the truth from yourself as well. Closet eating was a huge issue for me. I was like an alcoholic with a bottle in the woodshed. Mine was usually some potato chips under the seat in the car. Anyone who is obese can probably relate to the secretive eating away from prying eyes. The hiding of the evidence. I used to hide potato chip wrappers down the back of the couch, hide things in my desk at work. At home, I would eat a whole loaf of fresh bread in the morning, then go get another one to look like I hadn't. I think you get the picture by now just how I got so obese.

> **I even tried to help myself by limiting the amount of cash I had on me and sometimes left my wallet at home. I remember my wife asking me why I used cash and not my card all the time.**

I used to tell her I just liked having cash on me. No, I just liked having money that was not traceable to the amount of junk I was buying each day. I just did not want the number of times I ate fast food to be appearing on the statements from the bank. It would all be there in black and white then for everyone to see.

When I did eventually limit myself, and stopped carrying cash, this helped a lot. If you don't have that cash on you or access to cash, you can't feed addiction at the bakery or drive through. I know that sounds radical, but that really helped me in the whole process to be accountable. It is these little things that all add up when trying to change your mindset and form new habits. Trust me, I needed every little bit of help I could get, and I was looking for every edge I could get.

I was a prisoner of my problems with sugar and fast food and snacks. It had an iron fist grip on me I was almost resigned to the fact that this was me. I did not know it initially, but sugar was a much bigger problem than fast food for me and the harder of my addictions to beat. To beat a problem, you must admit the problem then find a pathway to resolve that problem.

> Denial for me was real. I lived in denial for years. I wasn't really a food addict. I was just was a tall big-boned guy. It was my genes.

Most of my family are overweight. I had every excuse going. Not owning up to my obesity and not taking control of my health was me living in denial. I was denying myself a life of wellness. Something had to change, and it finally did when I stopped denying I had addictions to food and started to address them. It is that initial internal war between a body craving the addiction and the mind trying to stop the addiction, and in my case, the body was winning, I needed to change that. I just didn't know-how. I had never investigated various ways to lose weight. I started to look around and watch some documentaries on TV that might help me. I am sure that is how most people start looking around for the answers to their weight problems.

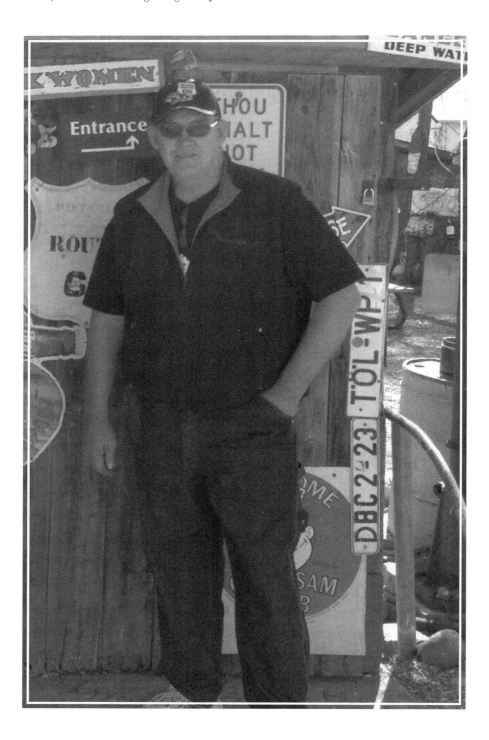

CHAPTER 2

2016 – More Diets, Some Success and Some Fails

In early 2016, I decided that juicing may be the answer after watching the Fat, Sick, and Nearly Dead documentary by Joe Cross, an Australian man who had some weight issues and made a documentary about traveling across America with a juicer in his car boot that he used to lose weight along the way. It made sense to me; I was not a big vegetable eater but I did eat a lot of fruit so I thought I would give it a go. I bought a machine and boxes of fruit and vegetables.

We were going to get married in Jan 2017, and we wanted to look our best for the big day. It was a motivation to do something. We had juices for breakfast and sometimes lunch, with a normal dinner with dessert. What a messy business that was. Looking back at it, I was making juices that were loaded with natural sugars from fruit. I know some people do well with it, but I didn't. Juicing was a pain for me. You always had to have mountains of fresh vegetables and fruit on hand daily. I got sick of trudging to the supermarket to get all the things that I needed.

It was messy and took a lot of time to prepare, so I soon stopped that. I just felt there was no way I wanted to juice for the rest of my life I needed something that was more sustainable, and I got sick of cleaning up all the sticky mess every day.

> **When I moved in together with my now wife, I started eating healthier meals at home and started going for walks regularly with her.**

Our diets were full of hidden sugar that we had no idea about, but we ate a lot more vegetables and salads than I was used to in my diet before we got together. Going for a walk was the first consistent exercise I had done in a long time and I hated the very thought of it. At first, I really struggled with walking. Carrying extra weight makes things so much harder. I was out of breath and struggled up the dreaded hills.

We probably only started walking for about twenty minutes, but we felt like we had run a marathon. I did get tired at first, but as we had a goal we just pulled on the runners before work, and off we went. Each time we went out, we got a bit further and faster. I started to get fitter and started to enjoy exercise more. I continued to do this consistently in 2016 and was making progress every day.

I knew the wedding was getting closer. There is nothing like a wedding to motivate you into action and I was on a mission to look as good as I could. Having this goal really focussed me on what I was eating and made me get out of bed to exercise. We both did it together which was great. I had a lot of weight to lose, and I was losing on average about

½ a kilo a week or a pound and had a few ups and downs as my food issues were still a big problem with breakouts frequent.

The exercise was getting some weight off, and my dream of wearing a decent cut suit when I married my forever girl was looking a real possibility. I had so many doubts and my food addictions were always present in my mental state. I tried to keep busy making the wedding plans and we took a quick trip over to Sydney to meet the celebrant and look at the wedding venue. I thought this was great as I had the big day coming up and wanted to look sharp. I was still hiding the fact I was a closet eater from my future wife, though I suspect she knew I was but never commented.

> **I was losing weight by having was lots of salads with fish or steak for dinner. For breakfast and lunch, we would have fruit and vegetable smoothies, made with almond milk.**

In hindsight, this also fuelled my sugar addictions. I just thought I was eating healthy food, not realising the high sugar content of the fruit in the smoothies.

By the end of 2016, I weighed 140 kg 308 pounds. That was a loss close to 20 kg (44 pounds) I was dropping clothes sizes and I was proud of myself. I was feeling much better than I did before when I was making no attempt whatsoever.

I was still very obese, but I looked better than I had in years. I did not look so slovenly, more like a guy who was an ex sportsman that had let himself go. I was still an imposing guy at 140 kg (308 pounds) and 6 ft 5 tall – no one was going to miss seeing me.

My toxic relationship with food was still there though, and soon enough, those drive-through trips became regular again as did my sugar binges at home. I was closet eating in my car, at home, or alone in my office. I am sure some of you resonate with what it feels like to be a closet eater or have an addiction to a food type. It sucks.

> **It started to become a real mental battle as I'd had a taste of improved health during that year. Owning up to my obesity was an important step in my journey, as was taking ownership of my weight and health and wanting to change.**

Finally saying to myself that I was a food addict and I had a problem was liberating. I had not ever looked at this part of my life critically. I was starting to think about what I was eating, rather than mindlessly eating everything in sight.

As I went to bed on New Year's Eve after a great night with Lou and her sister at a Balmain watering hole, I was excited about what the next year held. I was going to get more weight off and I was going to stop the fast food and sugar. I gave myself the usual New Year's Eve speech obese people recite to themselves around the world every year.

CHAPTER 3

2017 – Finding my Way to the Fasting Highway

A new year began with much excitement for me. I was to marry my forever girl Lou on Jan 29th, 2017. It was a stinking hot Sydney day and it was a perfect day in every way. My bride looked stunning and I felt like I looked okay too and was happy with myself. I had lost 20 kg (44 pounds) the year before, mainly by walking and reducing my trips to the drive-through and I was hoping it would continue. I was always hopeful.

Many people remarked how trim and well I looked. Yeah, right! I was still 140kg (308 pounds) and my height always made me look like I carried the weight well, but I was still a huge man.

During 2017, after the wedding that helped me focus on my health for a bit, I regained most of the weight back that I had lost in 2016. Not all of it, about 17 kilos (37pounds). Old habits die hard as I am sure you know about regaining and how frustrating that is. As an obese person, you are always on that constant roller coaster of weight loss weight gain. At least it felt that way for me, my whole life was a constant battle around food. I just never managed to get it under control and on an even keel. I would go well for a while, then the old ways would slowly creep back in. With the wedding and motivation over, my bad habits returned with a vengeance.

The visits to the drive-through became more frequent again in 2017 and the sugary treats and carb binges returned as well. I was blissfully happy in my life, but I just couldn't control my appetite for fast food and sugar. Regain is always frustrating no matter how small or big the regain is. Coming to the end of 2017 that regain of 17 kg (37 Pounds) really affected me.

> I thought I was getting on top of my addictions and here I was nearly back to where I started. I wasn't on top of anything, they were still there, and I was getting angrier with myself.

I just could not admit that I had a problem. I just didn't know how to overcome it at that stage.

I was not really walking much and had slipped back into all my old comfort eating patterns. After being so strict with the shakes and exercising regularly, I just couldn't make it stick and my old ways were back in place and the weight was creeping up again.

As 2017 was ending, we took a trip to Sydney to enjoy Christmas with my wife's family. I was nearing 157 kg (346 pounds). I had become lazy with my exercise routine and had not been motivated. I was not walking nearly as much as I was before the wedding and I was eating like it was my last day on earth again. I had no reason to do what I was doing. I was newly married, blissfully happy and work was going well. I was just still addicted to my issues with food and that was what was holding me back.

Apart from food, life was good, and I had the best wife ever whom I loved more by the minute.

> I used to eat when I was happy and eat when I was sad – it was never just related to one end of the range of my emotions.

I was looking forward to Christmas. My wife's family are all magnificent cooks and hosts they didn't disappoint that Christmas. As usual, the food was stunning and a lot of it. Oh boy, did I indulge in all my favourite Christmas treats. I stuffed myself silly for days. My mother in law made these incredible rum balls with an emphasis on the rum and I loved them. I would sneak a few every chance I got. I ate all the Christmas chocolate I could. I was revolting. My closet eating was reaching fever pitch and it was soul-destroying.

I was drinking a lot of alcohol that Christmas. I loved a beer, including a great all-day pub crawl around Sydney with my sister in law, which was an awesome, fun day. I arrived back to my in-laws in full flight, late for dinner, and not very popular with my wife.

A few days after Christmas 2017, Lou and I attended my lovely nieces› wedding in Wollongong or known simply here in Australia as the

Gong. As I put on my suit for the wedding on a very warm day. I really noticed how tight my pants were and how full I felt. It was a fun-filled wedding and my niece looked stunning. I indulged in a beer or ten to get the courage to dance like no one was watching. John Travolta, I am not but I do like to have a good time.

> **After that wedding, I felt so full and sick. I simply had reached the full level of my tank like so many times before. I had a very big tank, and this was a strange feeling.**

I had been stuffed so many times in my life with food, but this was a whole new level of full. I knew I had gone overboard with everything and feeling that full was next level for me. I had gone way too far, and I knew it, I just couldn't admit it.

I remember thinking how badly I had blown that good year in 2016 having lost some weight, only to regain most of it back in 2017. I felt like I had let Lou down badly. Of course, being the beautiful soul she is, nothing was said. Her love was always constant and flowed from her to me unconditionally. This meant a lot to me to have someone who was not judgemental of my eating behaviour that just loved me as I was. But it also let me off the hook and gave me a license to eat whatever I wanted without recrimination. I had no accountability and was back to my old patterns well and truly.

All of us have finished the year and thought, next year, I am going to lose weight to get healthy. Next year, next week, tomorrow I will start, and we just don't start. I am sure you are nodding your head up and down agreeing. Overweight people are the masters of procrastination and I was right up there in the gunner do this gunner do that category. I had started and stopped so many times with weight loss attempts they should have named a chainsaw after me. I remember lying in bed New Year's Eve 2017 thinking, "I can't do this, I cannot go another year as an obese man. Surely, I can beat this."

> "Tomorrow is a new year, and I am going to get healthier?" How many New Years have we all said that as an obese person?

It has been truly inspiring watching Graeme's journey unfold. It is just amazing. His dedication and discipline to retake his health is remarkable.

Rachel H., Western Australia

CHAPTER 4

The Start of My Journey

My mother in law is a very stylish woman had given me a gorgeous and very expensive David Smith shirt to wear home on the plane. I knew I was going to struggle to fit into it. I was not even close to doing up the buttons. I did what I usually did most Christmas days over the years. People would buy me 5XL and 6XL shirts that I could usually not fit into. I would put it in the too fat pile with the rest of the clothing gifts. I remember I was so embarrassed and totally annoyed with myself I was the size I was. I had to make an excuse for not trying it on and knew that the disappointment of those buttons not meeting was not something I wanted to share in front of my family. That shirt, as it turned out, played a very big part in my decision also to get this weight off once and for all. I was sick of having huge piles of clothes I just could not wear and hated the clothes styles that were in limited choices available to me because of my size. They just did not make me feel good.

I dreaded flying and had deep-seated anxiety around it. I was now tipping the scales at a whopping 160kg (352 pounds) and at 6ft 5, I was a very big, imposing guy. I was always grumpy about going to airports. I felt I would be publicly exposed and shamed in an economy seat not made for an overweight person my size. It was where my obesity really impacted me because I felt like I would be outed and ridiculed. It was my greatest fear – flying.

I had researched every plane model, every seat pitch to the inch so I knew which ones I could fit into. I knew which ones would sort of cope with my size. I was the master of the exit row. I knew every angle to get a seat that I could fit into and how to investigate the seating plan before booking.

I would show up hours before a flight just to get over my anxiety and make sure I got the best seats. Many beers were usually involved. People traveling with me hated it. I was revolting at airports like a child throwing a tantrum. People used to freak out when I walked down a plane aisle, with a look of, please do not let that fat person sit next to me. I couldn't blame them. I could see their look of horror as I stopped and indicated my seat next to them. They used to look up at me with dread and try to shrink more into their seats as I squeezed my way into my seat.

> **Everyone dreads someone spilling over onto their side of the seat and being way too close for comfort. It wasn't a very pleasant experience for anyone.**

Waiting to take off from Sydney to Perth January I, 2018 my anxiety levels were high. Sitting jammed in next to my poor wife, I felt so full from eating so much the previous week. Like it was right up to the top of my head full. I had really overdone the eating and drinking in that

Christmas week and had reached a new level of overeating that was something else, even for a seasoned overeater like me. I felt like I was going to explode in that very tiny economy seat that was clearly not made for a man of my size. I was in a state of anxious panic and felt that everyone was staring at me. Often when I flew, they were.

I looked across to my wife who was snuggling into me, smiling at me telling me, "it's OK. I am with you. Just breathe deep and relax and enjoy the flight honey", she said reassuringly.

> I thought right then at that moment in time I needed to get this weight off for once and for all so I could be around for this beautiful lady and live a very long life a life free of the burden of this crushing weight I was carrying.

That was it! The moment, for what single reason. I still don't know exactly why to this day; my mind just became so laser-focused on getting the weight off my body. Maybe it was all the times I had tried that came together to this one thought. For the next five hours on that plane back to Perth, I talked to myself in my head.

> Today is the day that I am done being obese. I was done being a slave to my weight and a victim of my compulsive eating.

Yes, I had given myself that speech over and over for forty years however, I had this beautiful lady next to me and I was taking up half her seat space. It was like, come on look at her she is amazing. She deserves better and deserves a man who looks after his health. I deserve it. How great would it be if I get this weight off? So that was the moment, on that day that I decided to take my health back once and for all. That plane trip was the catalyst that changed my life and forced me to address my addictions. I still had no plan, but my motivation was high, and I was making a commitment to have a go to finally rid myself of the weight that had hampered me my whole adult life.

CHAPTER 5

Learning About Sugar. The Awful Truth

My wife had bought a book at the airport on one of her business trips called "A life Less Sugar" by a New Zealand lady Amanda J. Tiffin. When I first read the title, I wondered what sort of weirdo would give up sugar. Why would you eat less sugar? Who does that? Surely sugar is not as bad as fat? That was how naïve I was. I swiftly threw it in the drawer along with my stash of getting fit, losing weight, becoming famous books. I forgot about it and I dismissed it without even reading it.

When we got home from Sydney, armed with my new motivation, I picked that book up again and started flicking through it. It had all these tables about how much sugar was in food, including hidden sugars and the story of this lady who had got her health back and lost a lot of weight by drastically reducing sugar and carbohydrates in her diet.

After reading the book, I could not believe how much sugar was in the food I was eating and was truly shocked. These were foods I ate every day, often at more than one meal. Most of my favourite foods were riddled with sugar. Now there is a surprise, I thought as I looked down at my huge girth. I was getting a picture of my problem. Sure, I knew the obvious high sugar content in some foods like chocolate, biscuits, and cakes, but it was the not so obvious hidden sugars that really got me. I was stunned that everyday foods were so high in sugar. I did not eat many of these things thinking that they were sugary food – to me they were just part of my diet. It was all laid out in a very easy to understand format and it made so much sense to me.

> ## Boy, did I have a problem with sugar, and I knew it.

Not just with the obvious sugary foods I loved but in most of the food in my pantry and fridge as well. I had made excuses for my issues with sugar and there they were staring at me right there in those sugar content tables. That book initially led me to investigate more about sugar and it became clear everything I ate, as in the most popular things I liked, were the root cause of my addiction to sugar and my obesity.

It soon dawned on me – Graeme, you're not just someone with a sweet tooth or who just likes a sweet treat, you are a full-blown sugar addict who needs to stop. I will never know exactly the amount of sugar I was consuming daily and I shudder to think of the actual real number. I ran a few rough guesses and it was up around 70-80 teaspoons of sugar a day. The WHO recommended intake for men is 8 teaspoons a day. I was having ten times that amount a day and that was scary enough for me to not even consider what those numbers would add up to over the course of a year.

I got interested in the foods I was eating and what was in them, and then I watched the documentary film "That Sugar Film", by Damon

Gameau about how he ate supposedly healthy foods that were high in sugar. It showed how sugar had affected his body over a period. That documentary really shocked me into action as I learned more about how it could affect you. The main problem I had was in the massive amount of hidden sugars in the food I loved to eat. One simple Google of other names for sugar showed me 56 different names for it. No wonder the average Joe can get confused looking at a label and think they are putting something healthy into their trolleys when they shop. Once I learned the common ones, I was able to spot them on the nutrition labels and leave them on the shelf.

> ## I started to look at the back of the packet when I went to the supermarket.

At first, it took forever to go around looking at all the labels. Many items that I would usually throw in the trolley were now off the table. Cereals and my beloved baked beans, they all had to go. My wife and I quickly learned that what we needed to eat lived on the outside of the isles and everything in the middle isles was pretty much a giant pile of sugar and carbs we needed to avoid. Many times, we were devastated to think that the food we loved couldn't come home with us anymore. Some days we were grumpy as hell and stomped out of the supermarket, wondering what the hell we were ever going to eat that tasted good and would make us happy.

Of course, over time we learned but those first few weeks were a killer, I will not lie. I got to the stage that if I couldn't work out what was in some food of the nutrition labels, I wouldn't eat it. From that moment on I just started visualizing the amount of sugar in the food, instead of seeing the food itself and that helped with the cravings. I soon started to not crave that sugary treat as the thought of the sugar content stopped me once I educated myself about what sugar was in what food.

Sugar goes by many different names on product labelling. The problem is there are just so many different names for sugar on those labels. Names that are not familiar to us make it confusing to work out what it actually is that is in the food you are eating. Here are just some of the major names used for sugar on the back of the foods you eat. After you learn these sneaky alternative names, one glance, and you will know what they mean, and what hidden sugars lurk in your food choices. I will list just a few of the other names for sugar. There are many out there. You can see what the consumer is up against.

Sugar by any other name.

1. Anhydrous dextrose	2. Agave
3. Agave Nectar	4. Beet Sugar
5. Cane Sugar	6. Cane Syrup
7. Carob Syrup	8. Castor Sugar
9. Confectioners' Sugar	10. Coconut Sugar
11. Crystalline Fructose	12. Date Sugar
13. Dextran	14. Fructose
15. Glucose Syrup	16. Glazing Sugar
17. Invert Sugar	18. Lactose
19. Maltose	20. Muscavado
21. Sucrose	22. Sorghum
23. Panocha	24. Powdered Sugar

After getting a handle of what foods were full of sugar like the processed snack type foods, I set about going through the pantry and fridge at home and boxed up all the foods that were very high in sugar content. There were things I loved, but they had to go. It really did shock me the high sugar content in some foods.

> **Foods that I thought were okay to have because they said low sugar or low fat was so wrong! If something contained more than two teaspoons of sugar per serve, I would look for an alternative.**

Things like tomato sauce that I had with most meals had to go. That was hard, but I was on a mission and knew if they were in the house, they were going to end up in me. One small dab of sauce was a teaspoon of sugar. I had a lot of dabs on my food, so the added sugar adds up. It was like sprinkling sugar on most of my meals.

To give you an example of just how much sugar I was accidentally eating because I had never looked on the labels, I will step you through one of my old breakfasts, so you get the picture. I used to eat a can of baked beans on toast a lot for breakfast. Depending on what brand you eat, there are 4-5 teaspoons of sugar in one can. Then, add in the orange juice I was also having every day. Again, depending on the brand, in one glass there are 5 teaspoons of sugar. Just to round off my sugar start to the day, I would often have a flat white coffee from the drive-through on the way to work that also had around 2.5 teaspoons of sugar before I added extra on top. So, what I thought was my healthy-is start to the day had already put up to 15 teaspoons of sugar in my body, and all before 9 am. No wonder I was addicted to the stuff.

> It just keeps piling up once you start to go through what you eat every day. Even in foods, you consider that are pretty good for you like yogurt with up to four teaspoons in a small tub of flavoured yogurt.

If you do have an issue with sugar and want to reduce it to get to your goal, then please spend some time learning to read what sugars are in the food you are having. Doing this was invaluable in overcoming my addiction to sugar. The World Health Organisation recommends that women should have up to 6 teaspoons a day and men 8 teaspoons of sugar a day for a healthy diet.

Once we had got all those high sugar foods out of the house, we started to replace them with higher quality products. We also shopped for food daily as we were always passing a supermarket. It was slow going at first in the isles because we had to read every label. After a few weeks, we had it sussed and realised most of our food choices lived on the outside isles of the supermarket and the stuff down the middle, as I mentioned was probably not going to help our cause. All the packaged foods were just so laden in sugar and we knew we would have to start cooking most of what we eat from scratch. Our trolley sure did look different – we looked like those healthy people! We were amazed at the different foods that we were buying.

We were able to access fresh food daily and not have piles of food in the fridge and cupboards. This was a great thing to do a shop more regularly and start eating that higher-quality fresh food. I didn't buy any soft drinks (or sodas) for the house, anything that was triggering my sugar issues was out. I just felt it was like learning about food for the first time. I had to learn over again the best foods that were for my body which I was going to get to my goal of wellness.

At first, we really struggled with the taste of all the low sugar alternatives. We were so used to eating sweet-tasting foods that the alternatives tasted bland and ordinary. Sometimes we cooked disasters that were inedible as we tried low sugar recipes. Sometimes even the dog turned his nose up at our efforts – you know things have changed if even the sausage dog turns down food. We also found some great ones that satisfied and surprised us. It really is trial and error to find food that suits you and how you like to eat.

> **Sugar is used in many foods to enhance the flavours. It is cheap and used to fill or change the flavour of food to make it more palatable.**

After a while, our tastebuds adapted to the new tastes, and now the foods I used to love taste excessively sweet to me. This still amazes me to this day just how much my tastebuds have changed and what sort of foods I now love to eat that are so much lower in sugar content. It really has happened to me – who would have thought it? Certainly not the old sugar addicted me before I started on this journey but it is so true.

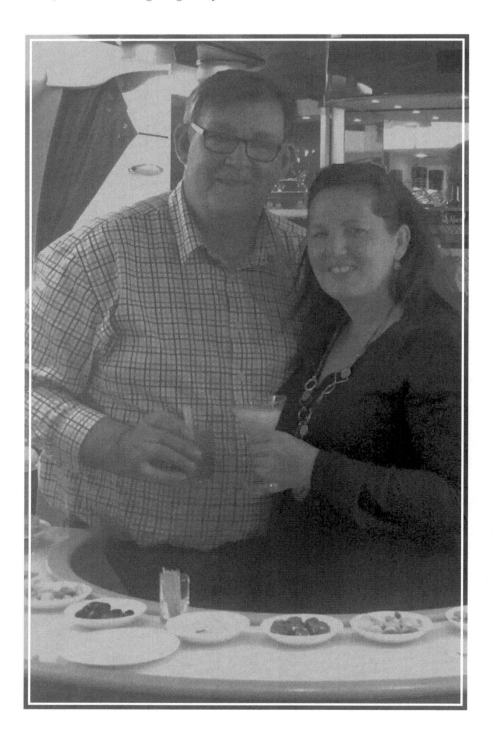

CHAPTER 6

Withdrawing from Sugar and Fast Food. My Cold Turkey Hell!

So, the cold turkey on my sugar and food addiction problems and my fight with obesity began early January 2018. There was no half measure for me to just ease into it. I saw no point. I had to be all in if I was going to beat this. I had to quit cold turkey and face my problems with sugar and fast food once and for all. I would urge anyone if you have an addictive issue with fast food and sugar, just quit it, draw a line in the sand and take it on head-on. Honestly, it was the best thing I could have done and one of the most unpleasant at the same time. Just cutting yourself off cold from lifelong addictions is not easy.

Now that I knew what was in all the foods I ate, it seemed ridiculous to keep eating them. I needed to do something about this now I had this more educated way of shopping for food and eating. I also knew it was going to be hell because of the massive amounts of sugar and carbohydrates I was used to having daily. There was no denying all the facts I had learned about why I was overweight and what was causing it, even if I had managed to lose weight in the past. It was time to face the music. I was ready. I knew that if I just reduced things a bit at a time, I was going to creep back to my old ways quickly. Full tilt seemed like a good option, but little did I know it was to be so difficult in the beginning or what sort of hell I was entering.

> **It was, without a doubt, the biggest battle I've ever had with myself. I fought through a brutal couple of weeks with withdrawing from vast amounts of sugar and fast food that I had been eating.**

When I say brutal, not in a painful way, just a spectacular battle of wills between my mind and my appetite. It was me against my problems with food. I was just so determined to bring an end my 40-year battle with obesity.

I never knew what to expect during the cold turkey phase. I had always quit and made excuses for why I could not continue and gave in to my problems with food and my out of control appetite every time. When I had tried diets or eating healthy before, I was still consuming spectacular amounts of sugar. I thought I was dieting but really all that hidden sugar was still sabotaging my weight loss every time. My cravings were always being met with hidden sugars in my daily food. No wonder I always failed.

For the first time, I was going to change that. I had no clue as to what was going to happen when I stopped cold turkey. Or the true extent of just how my food issues had hold of my mind and body. I just knew I had to stop. I had to do this hard core with no easing into it! Just STOP! I could stop myself from so many things – why was this any different? Then it dawned on me my problem was mindset – I knew I really needed to correct the way I thought about food. It was in my mind and I was ready for the fight to change that and to succeed.

During the first few days of cold turkey, it was not fun. I had the shakes, violent blinding headaches, and mental torture. I erupted with mood swings like I never had experienced before. I am usually a gentle guy, but this was out of the box. It was a like a 1000 people screaming at me 24/7 to eat that food, go get some sugar, go get a burger fries, and a shake. I was in serious hell. I had some wild dreams and it truly felt like something was inside me wanting to get out. I was in a fight within my mind and within myself. I started to find out what it was like to climb the walls of withdrawing from addiction that some poor people face with substances.

> **The first week was awful, to be honest. I couldn't function. I spent two whole days in bed with the doona over my head. I was withdrawing from every bad habit I had with food in my life.**

I would seriously consider taking leave from work when first withdrawing from food addiction issues and clear out your social schedule if you know you have been eating too much sugar and carbohydrates in your diet and you want to quit. Just lock yourself down at home and tell people around you this could get ugly. Apologize in advance for any snappy moments or for turning into something you are usually not. It is ok- trust me that the feelings are fleeting and will eventually pass soon enough.

> I was angry and it must have been hell for my wife living with me. I was snappy and I was awful, but I just had to get through it.

This line was well and truly drawn in the sand. I don't know what withdrawal from drug or alcohol addiction is like, but I sure found out what sugar and fast-food addiction withdrawal was like. It is important to note here that it is not that long before things get easier. That is important if you are thinking about cold-turkey or reading this going, "no way I'm not doing that, I'm just going to reduce sugar and cut down". That way, in my view, does not work for chronic addiction like issues.

Just stop, go through the withdrawal process, and get your mindset right. Start to take control. You can do it! Trust me if I did, you can, anyone can. In my view, if you want to address addictive behaviour with food you just must go cold turkey. You must just stop it the same as binge eating or grazing all day – just stop. You are the CEO of your plate. Legislate the plate and make a better choice for yourself.

I had already gone through the pantry and fridge, so everything in there was low sugar and low carbohydrate alternative. I did go and stare at my pantry and fridge often, as it was a habit, and did sorely miss seeing my old friends in there. It was weird at first to open the fridge and not see anything I really wanted to eat. That was strange –

there was food in there, but not the sort of food I would have usually grabbed with a smile. But I was on a mission. It really was a shock to me just how often I habitually went looking for food, for that sugar hit. At this stage I was still eating whenever I was hungry, just limiting my sugar and carbohydrate intakes to normal levels.

> **In those first few weeks, that was enough to turn me into one hangry man. I would eat something, and still go looking for a sweet treat to finish it off. It was just a habit.**

Or I would go looking for a bag of chips mid-afternoon. I knew there was no way I could have done those first few weeks without stringently clearing out every bit of sugar-laden food from my house and committing to this process.

Cold Turkey Starts Getting Easier

The withdrawal effects of sugar and fast-food addiction started to ease after about a month. I kept it up, and after about four weeks, I started feeling good. I had a feeling in my body that I liked, not the overfull, stuffed feel I craved before or that full stomach feeling. I was eating healthier food choices and finding alternatives with low sugar and low carb foods.

I started to eat lots of salads, meats, chicken, fish, lobster, and foods that didn't contain massive amounts of sugar. I had zero fast food and I could sense a turning point in my wellness journey.

I have tried to say just how bad those first few weeks were, and it was, but trust me, it does get much better. I was heavily addicted to sugar and fast food. Your issues with food may be nowhere near as bad and you may find it much easier – I was just full of sugar and it was not an easy time.

> **Banning myself from going to any fast-food stores or drive through seemed straight forward enough but the implementation in the early days of that ban was true torture and a battle of wits with bad Graeme and good Graeme.**

Some days I know the car would have just gone there itself if I didn't have an iron grip on the steering wheel. With some good food in the house sorted and a self-ban on fast food stores, I was getting there. I just told myself that they were off the table. I was not going to go through a drive-through for anyone or anything. I was done there. That was probably easier than my sugar cravings. I just stopped going to the fast-food stores, but sugar was an issue I had to sort out. Sugar was by far the worst of the two problems I had, for sure.

Looking back over my whole weight loss journey, it just made it easier in that I wasn't having the double whammy of adopting a new way of eating and fighting my addictions. I got the sugar under control first and then went on to intermittent fasting after the initial detox phase I put myself through to get rid of these addictions for good.

Detox from sugar and carbohydrates

My detox phase after the initial cold turkey went on for nearly three months, I had to make sure I had this beat. I used this time to find healthy alternatives in my food choices by experimenting with cooking and learning more about nutrition facts about foods. We sure made some disaster meals that tasted like cardboard but also found some gems that we still cook today. It shocked me when I found a good alternative that tasted good and was good for me.

All through my initial cold turkey, and subsequent detox period, the voices of my addictions were ever-present. As the days and weeks rolled by, they were, however fading though, as I became healthier. I felt well within myself, however, I was still very obese. I had lost about 15 kg 33 pounds in 10 weeks and was loving the way I was feeling and felt I really had come through the worst of it. The Cravings had gone away, and I started to taste food again and enjoy it.

> **It was amazing how quickly I did adapt to the low sugar diet from a taste point of view. It worked incredibly quickly really. The weight was really coming off me and I was loving how the scales were going down each day.**

However, I still had a nagging doubt as I continued this low sugar, no fast-food diet. We all know those doubts- the days when you go you think that you were happier when you were just an eating machine and very unhealthy. Is this all worth it? It so *is* worth it, trust me every step up the mountain is worth it to the wellness summit. Taking your health back is worth a couple of shitty weeks and it is worth the fight to do that. Sticking it out after that initial weight loss is hard when you know you have a ton more to lose but I was on a mission and nothing was going to stop me.

> **For the first time in my adult life, food was not controlling me. I felt I was breaking the chains of addiction that had dominated my life.**

I wasn't counting calories or macros. My theory was I had enough to track in my life and I just needed to eat cleaner. I was trying to get my head around some good quality food that was low in sugar and carbohydrates. I tried to limit my sugar intake to around eight teaspoons a day. I was able to do that by gaining the knowledge from researching nutrition labels and I had an app on my phone called Fat Secret which I could punch a food or product into and it would tell me the sugar carb and fat content.

From there I was able to keep under that 8 teaspoons of sugar daily. I also aimed for less than 50 carbohydrates in my food total per day, which was hard to do given some of the foods I was having. This helped me eat cleaner, healthier options, and helped get all the rubbish out of my diet. They say knowledge is power, and that is so applicable to food. Most of my life I had no idea what was in the food I was eating. I had no clue that those 99.9 percent of fat-free products were so high in sugars. I was feeling great and eating well and getting all the toxins out of my body. Now I just needed something else to kick me along.

I know this sounds like a pain in the neck, to check everything you are eating and, at first, when I started, it probably was. It took a bit of work to figure out what I could eat within those limits, but once I sorted it, I was on my way. After a while, I knew which foods were my friends and which ones I had to leave on the shelf at the supermarket. I simply didn't purchase what was not going to help me and this made it a lot easier for me. Your tastes will change after the first few weeks, and today my fridge looks completely different from before I started. The vegetable bin at the bottom of my fridge is full of overflowing now and the beer fridge now competes with sparkling water for space. We all know that is what we should be doing and eating but when you really get into it and really look at the labels it will change your world and that scale will start to move in the right direction.

I was having things like kale in shakes, keto style foods, lots of meats steak, pork, lamb, beef and salads, seafood, chicken, and deli meats like chorizo. I also ate lots of salami and cheese, low carb crackers with tomatoes and avocados, as I really like to have a snack board – anything that was low in sugar and carbs really.

> I avoided beer, bread, and chips, my nemesis foods. I was still eating a few times a day, but better-quality food and it was working for me. I started to feel good.

I have done a table here of some popular foods quantities that I used to eat, and often in more than the quantities listed, with their sugar and carbohydrates content so you can get an idea. I used to eat multiples of some of the serving sizes in the tables. This gives you an idea of just how much sugar I was consuming.

Food	Average Serving size	Number of teaspoons of sugar
Tomato Sauce	45g	3 teaspoons
Baked beans	220g	4.5 teaspoons
Yoghurt strawberry	170g	4 teaspoons
Banana	1	3.5 teaspoons (natural but still sugar
Flat white coffee	1 medium	3 teaspoons
Orange juice	1 cup	5 teaspoons
Strawberry jam	30g	4.5 teaspoons

Food	Average serving size	Carbohydrates
White bread	2 slices	25 carbohydrates
Big Mac	One Big Mac	35 carbohydrates
Pizza	1 slice meat lovers	28 carbohydrates
Potato chips	1 packet salted 100 grams	50 carbohydrates
French fries	1 serve	22 carbohydrates
Pasta	1 cup cooked	42 carbohydrates
Beer	1 can	12.7 carbohydrates

I just wanted to get a sustainable, long term health plan together for myself that I could follow easily and stick to for good. I had to look for a game-changer and that's when my life and health were about to take a life-changing turn for the better. They say winning the lottery is a big thrill – well what I discovered one day surfing the net it was like winning the lottery the day I discovered intermittent fasting. As it has turned out it has been the gift that has just kept giving.

CHAPTER 7

Hello, Intermittent Fasting Eureka!

People will often ask me how I came across intermittent fasting. Well, to be honest, it was purely by accident. In March 2018, I was taking a break from work on our property and scrolling on my phone looking for weight loss related sites on Facebook, as you do on a hot Sunday afternoon in the hammock! I came across this thing called OMAD. "What the hell is that?" I thought and searched for one meal a day lifestyle. Who does that? Are they crazy? You only eat once a day? That's nuts! Yeah, right, no one does that, it sounds like that's starving yourself. I dug a bit deeper about intermittent fasting as my curiosity about it grew. That led to finding the book Delay Don't Deny, by Gin Stephens.

I read the book description and thought, wow this sounds so interesting. What a great story, and I just liked the genuine explanation of it. I started researching more about intermittent fasting and it was like that classic light bulb moment. Eureka! I can do this plan. I reckon this can work for me. I got very excited I finally felt like I had discovered something very doable and that had some sustainability and some credible science behind it.

What I liked about intermittent fasting when I read about it was the sheer simplicity of it. Up until this stage, I was simply trying to eat healthier food and reducing my sugar intake per day. I am a simple guy with a busy life, so counting food calories or weighing food was never going to work in my life. I just didn't have time for that sort of thing nor wanted to do it. This seemed too easy to follow.

What is intermittent fasting?

I am just going to give a very simple, easy explanation as to how I started. What my fasting protocol was what I ate and how I put it all together. I'm sure you can find a 1000 things on the internet about the science around intermittent fasting. There is often a lot of confusing information for newcomers to fasting. It is one of the simplest things to implement but the mental part of it can be a challenge. You can talk about all the science in the world and that's important to do your own research or speak to your doctor about it.

> There really are only 3 steps to the actual process of fasting. You are fasting, eating, and then repeating that process daily – that is the foundation of it.

People who practice intermittent fasting stay in a fasted state for a longer period delaying when they eat each day. It gives our bodies and organs a good rest from digesting food and enough time to what I call "take out the rubbish". It also allows our bodies to burn through our fat stores which are not been fuelled by eating all day which in turn helps you to lose weight. Your body enters a state of ketosis because of low glucose from fasting allowing your body to use your fat stores rather than glucose. Autophagy is a self-cleaning process of your cells regenerating them in longer fasts.

> **Generally, the fat burning process really starts ramping up around that 18-20-hour mark from the research done.**

Intermittent fasting is also known as time-restricted eating and there are quite a few terms and more and more new ones that get coined regularly. Fasting has been around forever going back to the caveman days. Hunter-gatherers would go for long periods without food and there was no obesity epidemic. Everyone fasts, every single person who sleeps fasts. They go to bed and they are not eating, they are fasting during that sleep period which for most people 8 hours on average. People wake in the morning and the first thing most people do is have breakfast, it is named that for a reason, as you are breaking your fast after your overnight resting period.

> **The whole idea is to keep our insulin as low as possible during the fast and access our fat stores, then burn through them. Fasting also enables us to clean and regenerates our cells, and this is known as Autophagy.**

The Clean fast

A clean fast is where you only have black coffee, black tea, or water (plain or sparkling) during your fasted time. The clean fast is so important to be strict about, because as soon as you add any calories at all it will stop the process that you are trying to achieve. If you are adding things like cream in your coffee tea or milk or having diet soft drinks (or sodas), you are not fasting at all. When you add anything other than the four listed things you can drink, you spike an insulin response and your fast is over and you will not get the true benefit of the fast.

The magic happens in the clean fast. Get that into your mindset from day one and you will get the maximum result you can. We want to keep that insulin super low to maximize the benefits of the clean fast.

A dirty fast is where you add extra things into your fast. Some people will have cream in their coffee or a diet soda. You will probably get some weight loss results by dirty fasting, but they are not keeping their insulin levels low. By far, the better outcomes will happen from the clean fasting. I know this from reading thousands of testaments to that and living it myself.

> **Make that decision day one.
> I cannot recommend it enough –
> clean fasting is everlasting!**

With intermittent fasting, you simply clean fast, preferably for a minimum of 16 hours a day. You then open an eating window of a certain length, eat until you are satisfied, and then close that window. The message was that it wasn't what we ate, but simply delaying when we ate it. "Now that's a plan I want to try", I thought. I can do that.

I had already booted sugar and fast food out of my life and changed to healthier food choices during the detox phase. I did not want to change what I was eating as it was working for me. It had been a massive change in my life and a positive one.

> ## I was losing weight, feeling better, and didn't want to let all that work go.

As great as eating anything you want during an intermittent fasting window sounds, I had made the personal choice very early on for me that if I was going to do this and only eat one meal a day it's going to be window worthy. I really gave that a lot of thought about my food choices right from the start. I had started to change my relationship with food. Before I started the detox from sugar and fast food, I was coming from a place where I had made some poor choices daily many times a day for decades.

Now with intermittent fasting, I only need to think about food once a day. That was very appealing and really made my choices simple for the first time in my life. I just had to switch off my thoughts about food during the day – there were no choices to be made about what I was going to eat or not eat while fasting. There was no deliberating over food for a big portion of my day – I simply did not need to worry about it. For a simple, busy person this is great, as it is black and white. I found that easy after the first few weeks. That's the thing about fasting.

The longer that you do it the easier it becomes until it is just something that you don't have to think about.

Imagine being in a situation in your life where food does not dominate it? How amazing would that be? I had spent my whole adult life wondering what I was going to eat, it consumed my day, even when I had detoxed. It made me realise just how much food dominated all my thoughts. It was crazy when I thought about it.

> **I knew that I wanted to maintain everything that I had learned to this stage and then add this new way of living to see what happened.**

Sometimes you do have to restrict you do have to deny certain foods if you are trying to lose weight. I really took the delay takeaway as the main thing I wanted to focus on.

Addressing the problems, I had with sugar and fast food before I started intermittent fasting really helped me adapt to the fasting way of life much more quickly. It just made it easier than I was not having the double whammy of adapting to a new way of eating and fighting my food addictions together. I would strongly advise anyone who has problems with food like I did to try and get that addictive behaviour under control before starting intermittent fasting.

I was quite confident that, unlike other things I had tried, there was something very different about intermittent fasting. It was easy to understand, the rules were so few that I could get my head around it and start straight away. That suited me and my lifestyle. I had finally found something that interested me and seemed so easy and sustainable. I found someone in Gin Stephens and her groups that I really resonated with. That life-changing gem I had been looking for that had some long-term look to it.

When I started intermittent fasting, I simply determined an eating window time in a 24-hour period, and then I fasted for the rest of that time. You can decide do a 16-8 18-6 19-5 20-4 21-3 22-2 17-7 protocol – the choice is yours. The lower number is the length of time that you are going to eat. It is your eating window time. Sixteen hours is generally the recommended minimum amount of time to fast if you want to see some results from weight loss and other health benefits according to the research I had seen.

> I chose a 23-1 protocol, so a twenty-three-hour fast and a one-hour period where I took my one meal a day. I know, hard core, right? There was method in my madness.

What 23-1 meant was that I ate all my food for that day in that one-hour window. Initially, I thought if I only have a short time in which to eat, then I won't be eating and eating, and therefore with only one hour, I won't be able to get too out of control. Weird logic I know, but it worked for me. I also wanted to get the fat-burning time maximized after 18 hours and boy, did I have some fat to burn through.

When you first start, you can pick a window time that suits your home and work life and whatever length you feel comfortable with. If the idea of 23-1 which I chose to do is daunting and has you white knuckling, then you can try starting at 16-8 and see how you go with that. This means you are eating just after lunch, which is doable for most people when they start. It is important that you make this about you so stay in the comfort zone you are happy with. There is no rush, and you can tweak the experiment and swap out times to it works. That is the sheer beauty and flexibility of fasting. Start small and celebrate success and build from there. It is not a competition or a race, and you can change it as you learn what works for you.

> **The time of the day where you open your food window is entirely up to you too. You may be a shift worker and find that eating in the morning suits you better – go for it.**

For me, I like to eat early evening at the end of the day but can't eat late at night because I don't like going to bed on a full stomach. We tend to eat around 5.30-6pm. I also wanted to eat with my wife and family in the evening. You will find the window and time frame that suits you and your lifestyle. Just try some different times, and you will eventually settle on what feels right and gives you the results you want. Some people will constantly change their windows and eating times and that is fine too. Things happen, life happens, don't beat yourself up if you need to change it around to suit your family.

There is no more of an expert on your body than you, so you really need to decide what you feel you can cope with. That might seem strange to you at first. If you were like me, you have never listened to your body at all and have no idea what full or satiated or true hunger feels like, as you have eaten everything. Right from day one, you must have the mindset that you are doing this for you, so it must be all about you. You don't have to do super long fasts to start but aim for at least a 16-8 protocol to see how you go. Maybe try a 20-4 after you get used to it.

> **You will be so proud of yourself and realize that food is no longer in the drivers' seat of your life.**

Find that sweet spot that works for you. Some very experienced people I know found a 19-5 protocol worked for them. It really is great that having the flexibility to move that fasting protocol around until you do find that sweet spot your niche fasting eating times. Try it, change it, tweak it was my motto. It turned out 23-1 worked well for me so I stuck to that right through the weight loss phase, with a few exceptions. I was on a mission the weight had to come off.

Graeme has passed on his knowledge of intermittent fasting to me and it helped me lose more than 25 kg (over 50 pounds). Graeme's thoughts around mindset and helping troubleshoot my issues has been fantastic. Watching his inspiring transformation motivated me to start intermittent fasting and it has changed my life.

Luke M., Esperance, Western Australia

CHAPTER 8

My Intermittent Fasting Protocol Step by Step How I Started

Step 1

I clean fasted for 23 hours a day from day one most days I opened my window at 5 pm

During my 23 hours of fast, I did not eat anything. The only beverages I consumed were:

> Black coffee or black tea or water –
> still or plain sparkling.
>
> That was it. I had nothing else during
> my fast to keep it clean.

I initially chose 23 hours as my fasting period as the research had shown the benefits of fasting really started to kick in around the 18-20-hour mark. Your body starts accessing your fat stores and the magic happens with so many other aspects of your health as well. As I mentioned, you pick a window and a fast time that you are comfortable with to start. This is going to be a lifestyle and it needs to fit in with daily life, and you can always change it up down the track once you get the hang of things.

Step 2

I had a one-hour eating window with a snack plus my main meal, then sometimes dessert. I have a couple of coffees with cream during that hour and eat until I am satisfied. Then I close my window. I always think of it as going out for an evening meal where you have a three-course dinner. Most days, I think my actual eating time might only be 20-30 minutes over that hour. It is quick and lets me get on with the rest of my evening and not think about food again.

> **Astoundingly, I found that intermittent fasting cured my insatiable appetite. I simply got to the stage where my previous ferocious appetite was corrected, and much, much less than it was.**

You will find this as well as you go along your own journey. Satiety signals that you have never noticed before will arrive toward the end of a meal and you will learn to listen and say to yourself, "ok, that is enough for me now. I'm good for today". That is a profound thing for a guy who had no off button or did not even know what feeling full meant.

I discovered that I really didn't need as much food a day to sustain myself which was a wonderful surprise to me. If you put all the food that I ate in a week on a table compared to what I eat now, it would be shocking. The difference in volume would be shocking, but also what I eat as well. Looking back, it was probably about four weeks in that I noticed that my appetite was starting to correct itself which was so amazing and delightful to me. This was working!

How did I know when I had enough in my window? I listened to my body when I got that full feeling, I stopped. I didn't keep going until I was stuffed, just satisfied. After a while, the satiety levels are automated as appetite correction kicks in. So, whatever you're eating window try to eat till you feel full and satisfied, and then stop. Try not to get to that stuffed feeling, just a satisfying feeling.

> **It is important to note, whatever the length of the eating window you just don't keep eating the whole time over that 1-2-4-8-hour period.**

Eat until you reach satiety. Eat mindfully and take your time to listen and reach that full level and stop. These feelings will be signals that perhaps you have never experienced or listened to before. Our bodies will tell us amazing things about regulating what we do if we just take the time to slow down and really notice what is happening when we eat, rather than mindlessly stuffing food in our mouths because we think we have to at certain times of the day. If you have a longer window, try, and listen to these signals. After a while, they will happen, and you will be amazed that you are leaving food on your plate.

Step 3

Repeat steps 1-2 again the next day. Wash-rinse-repeat!

That is all I did 7 days a week for the first 16 months on intermittent fasting every single day. Once you start it with a plan you do just put it on autopilot, and once you have a protocol that works for you and it becomes part of daily life.

> **For the first week or so, you will find it weird that you just simply don't eat for a large part of the day.**

Those habits of a lifetime are firmly in your life, and it takes a few self-checks and a detour of the kitchen to keep going. If you are finding it tough, go do something that will distract you or keep your mind off the fridge. I often found that I would distract myself right before my window opened as I was struggling a bit, only to find that I actually ended up extending the fast for that day because I got busy and forgot about food. That signal to eat three times a day will eventually fade more and more, and you will find that it doesn't even feature in your daily thoughts anymore.

I know the steps sound very simplistic and that is because they are. That is the true beauty of intermittent fasting – it really is that simple in its implementation. It is also adjusting to the mental side of doing it and rethinking how you relate to food. That is where mindset kicks in. How do you get in that space mentally that you are only going to eat once a day when everything goes on around you and people are eating everywhere? Trust me, after a while you don't even give that a second thought. Those around you eventually just accept that is what you do each day. Just stay the course and others will adapt and accept this is what you are doing.

My advice is to try not to over complicate things in the beginning. Keep it simple and don't spend all day trying to analyse science. You are an experiment of one, so just pick a fasting protocol that suits you and your life give it a go. Be prepared to tweak as you go until finding a protocol that works for you. It is not a complicated health plan at all, and nothing could be easier or simpler. There are just three steps. Fast, feast, repeat.

> **You need to make this sustainable. It's not punishment. I chose to deny some foods, but many people who are intermittent fasters just eat what they crave in a window once a day and do very well.**

There are people out there who live on junk food in their windows and still lose weight! Lucky people They may lose slower than someone who eats a clean whole food type window. There is no rush and there is no competition. For me, I like the health benefits I have had from eating less sugar and no fast food, so I have stuck to that. This is your journey how fast you want it to go on it is up to you. We all have time. Above all else make it sustainable for you. You will work out how much food you need to sustain your body daily and you will also learn to listen to your body. Once you are full, stop and close your window. Just because it is a 2-3-4 hour eating window does not mean that you must eat that whole time.

What I eat during my eating window

Everyone always wants to know this. Yes, but what did you *really* eat? Like it will be some sort of amazing combination that will help them lose weight. I can tell you that I simply follow intermittent fasting and eat a low sugar diet with not too many carbs. When I started, I really thought about food choices more carefully for my window and make sure that it was not wasted on something crappy. I realized early on it had to be window worthy, after all, it is only once a day and I prepared my food. I had waited all day for this one hour, and I was going to make it as good as I could.

> I started plating things up with nicer presentations to make it fun. I really appreciate now that food is as much as a visual experience as anything.

I try to make what I am eating visually appealing. I usually put my snack on a nice board. This is a lot different than the brown paper bags of the drive-through on the way home where I would not even look at the food I was eating and just tried to shove it down as quickly as possible. I am no chef, but I do like to make my food look as appealing as possible. I like doing this extra preparation, and it is not a chore as it is only once a day.

I usually opened my window around 5pm on most days with a snack rather than go straight on to a big meal. I often had a plate of cheese, crackers, chorizo, and tomatoes first. I am a creature of habit, so my snack each day was mostly similar. I still eat cheese and crackers most days as a snack opener as I just love it.

> **When I first started there were a few things that were in my favour when choosing foods for my main meal, as I love seafood, meat, chicken, and eggs which are all low in sugar and carbs anyway.**

We have a lovely big vegetable patch and I liked the salads we grew in our garden, so I was able to have a huge variety for my main meals without all the junk food I used to eat as a food addict. I do not weigh or count anything like calories or macros. I had enough to track in my life with family and work. That's one of the great things that appealed to a fasting lifestyle. I didn't have to track food -I just knew it had to be better food. Do you see the difference?

People often say you become a total food snob after a while doing intermittent fasting. I agree totally with that. It feels good that my tastes have changed. It's amazing, and it was such a shock to me that I just had no desire for unhealthy food, after a few weeks of intermittent fasting. I felt I really had turned the corner. I was becoming one of those people who made the salad choice when out to lunch or dinner.

I started to go to places where the food was better quality and had low sugar and carbohydrate options. I happily chose healthier options on the menu rather than go for the sugar-laden ones. Wow! I then stopped thinking much at all about food during the day which was a huge non-scale victory for me. Food once dominated my mind all day every day. I am pretty sure I dreamed about burgers, fries, chips, and pizzas when I was obese. It was surprising how quickly all this happened and how differently I felt about eating food.

My main meals became more nutritious as I got deeper into my fasting journey and I got more creative in the kitchen. Ok, I may have nearly burnt the house down and destroyed the oven that one time the rugby was on and I forgot about what I was cooking, but I was learning! What you have in your main meal, however, is entirely up to you.

> **Eat what you crave, see how it pans out for you then tweak the choices as you go.**

You could be one of those lucky people that can eat anything you like and make intermittent fasting work. These people do exist and I am sure we are all a little jealous of them. Just give it a go if you aren't one of those lucky people, examine what your food choices are for your window and adjust. It's a real trial and error situation at the start. Just make sure you maintain your fast.

You can chop and change whatever you like to find your sweet spot that works for you. I haven't had any fast food from a chain store for two and a half years now. I still have the odd homemade pizza or homemade kebabs now and again. I also have things like our own burgers at home. If I am out, I tend to go for the meat options with lower carbohydrates like a steak and salad.

At home, we have things like nachos, casseroles, and a lot of soups in winter that are all home-cooked from scratch, so we know what is in them and they aren't riddled with high sugar sauces. I am sometimes still amazed at how this food transformation has happened, as I never thought in my wildest dreams that I would be that guy who preferred the healthy options on a menu. I am living proof that it is possible to rewire how what sort of food you naturally want to eat each day. and I am sure you will be amazed too when you start.

> **I do have a dessert most days.**
> **My kind of dessert would consist of some**
> **strawberries and blueberries with some**
> **Greek yogurt and a coffee with cream.**

Sometimes I would have a cheese board for dessert to close my window. It just depended on the day. I probably had a dessert more on the weekends when relaxing and I have a coffee or two with cream every evening. It just all depends on how full I feel after the main meal.

I was a very big social drinker and loved nothing better than a party around a keg. It has been a huge part of my social life. Beer just affected my weight too much in my life, and it was one of my triggers that would spike my weight and make me reach for the chips. So, I knew that I would have to avoid it, just like fast food. Beer and chips go together for me, two of my biggest problems. I just knew I would have to let it go to get through this and start to get healthy. I was so focussed on getting to a goal, that I knew that if I got on the beers, all that focus would go out the window in one sitting, so I decided to avoid it. I am sure most of my mates thought I was crazy, to begin with. Where had the party boy gone? Now they don't even comment.

> I really didn't drink much alcohol at all through the first year of my journey. If I did, it would be a vodka and soda water, but I laid off the beers.

I used to drink gallons of diet sodas every day and giant milkshakes featured in all my fast-food orders. I stopped buying both and the beer fridge got filled with sparkling water instead. I mainly just drank water or sparkling water on most days in my window. I was on a mission. In my window, I would have one or two coffees, long black with cream. Sometimes I will have some green tea or black tea as well, both in my window and when I am fasting, but I really am a coffee bloke. I have bought several nice coffee machines and look for quality coffee when I am out and about now. That is so different from my instant coffee days. I can really taste the difference now and appreciate a good barista!

The Food Snob I became through intermittent fasting

I never thought I'd become a food snob but here I am a full-blown food snob, hands in the air admission. It was pretty apparent very early on that I was becoming choosy about what I ate. I go by the mantra that if I am only eating once a day it must be good it has to be window worthy or it's a waste of a good once a day meal.

I started finding I was choosing things my body needed rather than the addictive, high sugar food that I used to eat. Lovely food now attracted me – the fresh highest quality meat, the best seafood, awesome cold cuts, and fresh salads.

The foods I used to crave and eat in huge quantities like chips, bread, pies, cakes, and fast food were just not on my radar anymore. I had transformed, not only my body but also my mindset. I had transformed my whole relationship with food, and I became a food snob instead of a food addict. It's all about making the right choice for me and you will find what suits your food-wise. You may well start eating all the things you usually do, then, as you live this lifestyle longer you may gravitate towards a higher quality type food. At the end of the day, there is that word choice that is what is so freeing about this lifestyle.

How do you not offend people when you are a food snob or just want great food if you are at a function or a work social or invited to a friend's place for dinner? You tell them the truth and tell them what you do and why you do it. I sometimes eat something before I go to a function if I think the food will be ordinary. That way I simply say, "I'm good thanks I had something before I came". No one will question you if you say you already ate and are full. Work functions are easy, it's the going to a friend's house that's been baking all day that is a bit trickier. Most of my good friends know I fast so they won't push the issue. Often, I will say that looks so good is it ok if I make a plate up and take it home to eat later.

Most people respect that I am an intermittent faster and now my daughters arrange our coffee meets around my window – how good is that!

The only thing that disturbs me about being a food snob is that I became a bit too judgemental of others' shopping trolleys or people's food choices. I had to really check myself and tell myself not to judge others at the supermarket with a trolley full of junk food and obese kids with them. It breaks my heart to see that, but they need to find their own way to wellness it's not for me to stare or lecture.

> I am just glad keeping my eyes on my own plate allows me to decide what is on there for my meal. So, I can deal with the tag of food snob, it is a lot better than a tag of morbidly obese.

I just don't want to waste an eating window. It's so annoying when I do that. I look at the very foods that used to dominate my life when obese and cringe when I see them. I just have no desire to even look at them let alone crave them. Been able to taste the joy in food now has been huge for me. Before it was just food consumption, I really enjoy my window and savour what I eat take my time and enjoy it.

Appetite Correction – It's a Thing

We often hear the term AC or appetite correction talked about a lot in the intermittent fasting community. Well, my appetite needed a lot of correction that's for sure. When I was detoxing from sugar and fast food first ten weeks of my journey, I still had a big appetite. I was just eating cleaner foods and losing weight, but my appetite was still strong.

After about three months into my intermittent fasting life, appetite correction started to happen for me. To circle back a bit, in my old days, I could eat two large pizzas easily by myself or a whole loaf of bread and be looking for another one in a day. One of the things I loved about intermittent fasting was that you eat till you are satisfied then stop when full. After a while, I learned that eating to satiety was a thing it really was that art of mindful eating. When you get to that moment, you start listening to your body and it tells you that's enough time to close that window now.

It changed my whole mindset about what amount of food I needed to sustain my body daily. It's quite amazing what little food we do need. We are told all our lives we need to eat three meals a day plus snacks and if you skip breakfast you will have no energy. Breakfast is the most important part of the day and you must eat five fruits and five vegetable types – you all have heard that in life no doubt. We had that drummed into us constantly when I was growing up in New Zealand.

Well, I think that myth is well and truly busted these days and I think we were duped by the food industry and clever marketers. What appetite correction has done for me is that it has allowed me to savour my food more. To truly savour the goodness of food was something I never did when obese. I was just in a hurry to stuff as much as I could in without enjoying it. I just wanted volume as much as I could eat until I felt ill.

> **I have lost count of the number of times I have exercised fully fasted first thing in the morning and had so much energy.**

No sign of hunger at all or that feeling I must eat something I am hungry. I just did not have that same hunger or desire for food. Right there was appetite correction in action it's a real thing with fasting.

> **I can't even imagine waking up now then having a big fry up or a giant bowl of cereal to start my day now. It is not something I want to do or crave to do. It's amazing how my life was so dominated by food but now through intermittent fasting, it is not.**

If I want breakfast type foods, I just have them in my evening window and that's what I love about the flexibility of this way of living.

My appetite fully corrected I think after about three months of fasting. It really was great to learn that I didn't need mountains of food all day to sustain myself and that one meal a day is more than adequate. I never thought anything would correct my previous massive appetite. I get full quite quickly now, I just reach that satiety point and stop, and I am sustained for that day. The next fast begins and so it goes on, and quite soon you don't even think about your fast you just do it as part of the day. The day you wake up not thinking about food or hungry you are as a food addict is a day you know appetite correction is starting to kick in.

Cost of fasting

I don't know that it saves me a lot of money intermittent fasting, apart from not buying so much junk food and buying coffees. I probably did save some money by not going through the drive-throughs every day that's for sure.

My value on things changed a lot after beginning fasting. I started to want really good quality food and today, my days of cheap cuts of meats and poor-quality processed food are long past. It gets back to that mantra that I followed from the beginning that something I eat must be window worthy. I would much rather pay twenty-five dollars for a decent steak to have in my window than buy a seven-dollar value meal at the fast-food store. I find I now spent more money on higher quality food the best cuts of meat and I would also buy expensive fish and other seafood. I just want quality and that can cost more than processed foods I used to throw in the trolley.

So, I really don't think the savings from intermittent fasting in general shopping is that much. Whatever I was saving from the food I was spending on clothes and shoes. To be honest the only big money that fasting has cost me really is new wardrobes and I am totally down with that. I think savings on food bills balance out somewhere else. Please don't do fasting because you think it's going to save you some money. Do it for health reasons.

> **I don't have to buy premium economy seats or business class seats now to travel as I can fit into normal seats now.**

I will always be tall though, so I usually try to fly in the pointy end when I can. It is a great feeling that my weight does not dictate my seat on the plane anymore.

I often used to think when obese if I died how embarrassing would it be to be for my family for me buried in a piano case and hire a forklift to lift my coffin. That might sound morbid but at 360 pounds it costs a lot extra for a funeral with the logistics around that. I am also sure I will have saved all the medical bills that were associated with my health issues that have now disappeared.

The 15 steps to self-examine if you on the struggle bus with Intermittent fasting

These fifteen questions may be useful to go through if you have been trying intermittent fasting and have reached a bit of a stall, or things aren't working for you. Sometimes, we need to really get to the bottom of things, and asking the hard questions are tough. Be gentle with yourself, maybe write down the answers and then pick them up again the next day and see if you feel the same or your answers would be the same.

1. **What's my biggest barrier to me doing intermittent fasting?**

2. **Do I feel like I am addicted to food sugar alcohol is there a trigger holding me back?**

3. **Am I under a lot of stress? Am I eating because of stress or need what is causing my stress?**

4. **What will life look like for me without this weight? What will I be able to do in my life that I can't do now? What will I be able to do so much better?** This is hugely important and helps to visualise in your mind what you aim to do without the weight on your body.

5. **Do I waste energy comparing myself to others?** If I am, I need to stop -comparison is the thief of joy. This is my journey I'm, doing this for me. You need to stop comparing to others. You are unique, comparison is futile and soul destroying and you are the experiment of one.

6. **Am I committed to doing this for me and only me?** Am I treating this as just another diet to lose weight not a lifestyle change? Rid yourself of diet mentality and focus on a change of life style in the way you eat.

7. **Why can't I relate to what I read and hear about intermittent fasting? What are the stumbling blocks? Am I afraid of something? What is nagging away at the back of my mind? Why isn't the information convincing me?**

8. **How long did I give it a real go?** You need to give this time a minimum 6-12 months then do a self-critical review. A few days weeks or a couple of months is not long enough to see real results and all the health benefits that could be yours.

9. **Am I dirty fasting?** Are you strictly clean fasting with water, black tea, coffee or plain sparkling water? If you are having anything other than those four things in your fast you are simply not fasting you are just calorie restricting.

10. **Am I binging in my window or eating to satiety? Am I eating to fuel my body or am I eating because my window is open for another hour even though I am satisfied and full?** Learning to eat to satiety may take a while but is crucial to long term success. It will happen – that moment when you go enough is enough don't eat past that point.

11. **Could my food choices be better?** If this isn't working for you, the answer may be in your food choices. **Do I need to restrict anything to I get to my goal is the question?** This is really a case of trial and error in the beginning. For example, some people are profoundly affected by things like carbohydrates or alcohol that may spike their weight while others can consume these things and still lose weight. Finding out those trigger foods and working out what affects you will really help you to stay the course and get where you want to go at a steady rate.

12. **Do I need to find a mindset coach or experienced mentor to help me?** Some people respond better to that one on one coaching or mentoring or a step by step course. Personally, looking back, I would have gladly paid a coach or mentor for some advice particularly around the mindset. Yes, you can get all the information for free you need but an experienced coach can help you through things at the right time. Reading a book is one thing but learning to apply what you are reading is another. This is where a coach can help some people.

13. **Have I seen any changes at all health wise since I started?** It is not all about the weight loss. **Have you seen any changes at all to things like mental clarity, the way you feel, or any changes in the way your clothes fit?** Any changes to your skin any changes to inflammation. **What are your energy levels like? Have they increased?** You may just be focusing on the scale and not seeing these changes happening.

14. **Have I honestly applied myself and committed to this? Am I moving at all? Am I doing any exercise?**

15. **What will my life look like if I don't do this for me? If I don't get healthier what impact will that have on my partner my family, my life, and my future? How will it impact on me in later years?**

Obesity is a hard life and a miserable existence compared to been a normal healthy weight. Yes, intermittent fasting can seem hard but so is being obese and its hard on your partner and family if your obesity shortens your life span

> **Within these answers, you may find the key that helps you understand why you are not as successful with intermittent fasting as you would have hoped.**

All of your frustration with intermittent fasting may be right there on the page and it may just give you a key to your future success. You may need some help, or some more information about some aspect that you need to tweak.

The key thing is not to compare or expect the same results as others as we are all different. You are the experiment of one and you will find success on this fasting highway if you give it a good go.

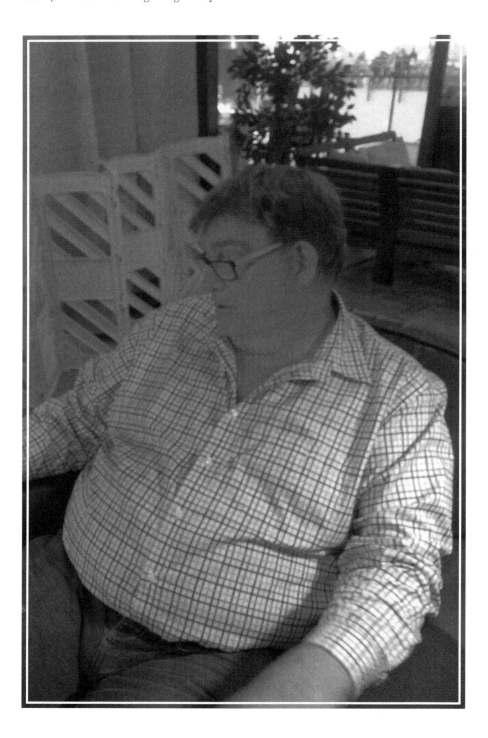

CHAPTER 9

Mind Set – Getting Your Head in The Game

My mindset around all this new way of life was something I worked on a lot and it was such was a crucial part of my journey. My focus in my work or organizing my business, home, and family matters was always good. I just needed to apply those principles to my lifestyle change with food and adapting to intermittent fasting. That sounds like a simple idea, but it is laden with all sorts of traps and pitfalls if you don't really sort out how your mind is going to affect what results in you can get. Anyone overweight has been sabotaged at some stage from their own mind who takes over the desire to lose weight and derails it with food.

When I first started, I didn't tell anyone except for my wife. It did sound like an extreme way of life, and I knew that I would get some ribbing about it. I thought, if this works, I am just going to let my results do the talking for me. There was that fear of failure lurking there again and the fear of the unknown. Somehow though, deep down, I just had this feeling that intermittent fasting was my jam. I just knew that I had to overcome my addictions with food, or I was destined to a life of obesity and likely an early grave. I just never had the right mindset with past diets. I knew that had to change with intermittent fasting and it was game on.

> **In the past, I had always told everyone I am starting a diet or on a diet and usually, it was met with a raised eyebrow and an "Oh, another diet Graeme? yeah right".**

I had tried all sorts of weird and wonderful diets in my life-you name it and I tried it. I had success a few times, but I would always pile the weight back on and then some for good measure.

I think for me, the beauty of it all, was that I tackled my addictions to sugar and carbohydrates first before I got into fasting. It really got my mindset into a positive state before I started my fasting journey. intermittent fasting is not a diet, it's a lifestyle. That's the first thing to focus on. That is important to get rid of that old diet mentality. There were no counting macros or calories on the path I was following and that was great for me, it was simple. If you do want to do that though, go for it, but for me was something I didn't want to do. I just needed to eliminate the foods that didn't work for me in my eating window. The very foods that had made me so obese in the first place.

I was rewiring the way I thought about eating and when I ate. I wanted to train myself in mindful eating and learning to enjoy eating slow deliberate and making my window an enjoyable experience each day.

For most of my life, I was told to eat three meals a day plus snacks to be healthy. It was ingrained in me by my parents that breakfast was the most important meal of the day and that I needed to eat lots of fruit and veggies. We have all had them parroted to us over and over all our lives or in mainstream media. So how do you get past that? How do you rewire your thinking? How do you go from having three meals a day and snacks mindset to one meal a day? It really is an internal process that only you can change in yourself. For me, it was an easy recipe to follow. Eat. Don't eat. It was black and white and crystal clear. Not counting calories or tallying up food each day was so refreshing.

When I started this weight loss journey, I often wondered how I was going to stop punishing myself mentally about my food issues. How often do we hear about people who express shame and really beat themselves up about overeating? I used to have a buffet regret nearly every day of my adult life mainly because I was sickly full of food that I knew was killing me but that I reached for every day, most of the time.

I hated the feeling and really made myself miserable but continued to do it before I found the way out. It is a terrible cycle that happens to so many of us. That inability to just say no is so hard to do, and the crushing punishment and self-loathing that we inflict on ourselves afterward is so debilitating in all aspects of our lives. I wanted to desperately change that.

> **I knew that I needed to flip my thinking and start celebrating the small wins I was having.**

I started thinking more positively and quit being such a critic of myself. I started loving myself first. That was so crucial to everything I was doing. I started to look in the mirror each morning and tell myself I was ok rather than beat myself up with toxic thoughts about my failures with food control. This was something that I had never done before. It was new, and some days I sure didn't believe my little internal dialogue in front of the mirror, but I kept at it. As the weight started to come off, I started to truly believe it as well.

> **When I discovered intermittent fasting Facebook groups I was amazed blown away and totally engrossed in reading all the stories and the before and after pictures were mind-blowing.**

I was like wow, you know what? If these guys can do that, so can I, and am going to do it! I could see the determination on their faces and read the mindset focus on the posts. These were real people who had struggled just like me and turned their health and weight around. They all did it in different ways but every one of them was raving about the weight and health success they were having. I was hooked. These were not just people who needed to lose a few kilos, they were big sizes and they had managed to get some spectacular results.

I drew up a list of my goals and what life was going to look like without this weight. I wrote down all the things I would be able to do when I get to my goal. Every silly thing I could think of that I had not been able to do in the last 30 years went on that list. I think that putting pen to paper really makes it a bit real, and it is good to go back and see what you can do as you get fitter and start to lose weight. Things that I thought were impossible I am now doing regularly in my life. I look different, but I feel so different on the inside. My inside dialogue is a whole new me too.

My initial goal was to just stick to fasting for a year and see what happens. This was a lifestyle change for me, and I needed to give it time. My mindset with that was it's taken me fifty-five years to get this obese it's going to take time to reverse that. I knew I was not in any hurry and had to trust the process, make the clean fast part of my day, and tweak my food choices and window length until it worked for me. I had always looked at diets as a short-term thing before – if I diet for this long, I will be this weight.

> **This was a totally new way of looking for a thing for me. Once I got my head around the lifestyle concept, the idea of going slowly didn't worry me. I was in this for the long game.**

If you do the same thing, you will be on your way in no time. Some people will have spectacular results and others will be slow turtles. I know my wife is a turtle and that really makes her mad that I wasn't. More than once she has stomped down the hallway after getting on the scales, but she realizes this is a lifestyle, not a diet, and keeps going.

My whole thinking about life changed. My new thought process was to eat to live not live to eat. As I was getting healthier, and my mental clarity got sharper, it allowed me to get into a great mindset. The way I thought about myself and how I walked through the negatives that popped up from time to time was great. Tell yourself over and over you can do this. No one has ever died because they skipped breakfast or lunch or both. Hunger is a state of mind it is not an emergency. What is better, a life of obesity or delaying when you ate food in your day? That's how I looked at it.

Staying active in Facebook groups helped too as it was a positive vibe and I was feeding off the success others were having. It really drove me. These people were my jam, and it was so important for my mindset to engage with people on this same journey. I started to chat with other people who were just starting like me, people who were halfway through, and veterans who had been maintaining for years and living a fasting lifestyle.

> **Surround yourself with likeminded people if possible, ask a friend or a colleague to be an accountability partner. Join some fasting groups or come to my group on Facebook, The Fasting Highway.**

I had never been much of a person for joining groups online before but reading similar stories and seeing other big size people have amazing results really lifted me up. I celebrated my wins and people cheered me on. It was something that I had not had a lot of in my life and it felt great. Whatever you choose to do, stay strong, stay focused, and those negative thoughts in your life don't have to live inside your body. Make the decision from the outset to do this for you and whatever anyone else says, just do you.

CHAPTER 10

The First-year Summary of my Journey with Intermittent Fasting

Summer 2018 rolled around, a year into my intermittent fasting journey, and it was time to head over to Sydney again for Christmas with my wife's family. I was a very different looking man to the one that wobbled in a year ago. At this point, I was down nearly 50 kilos or 110 pounds. There were a lot of shocks and a lot of disbelief a lot of what the hell when I walked in. I was so happy and excited to show them how I looked. They were all gobsmacked, and their reaction floored me a bit and I started thinking I had something wrong with me. My mother in law thought I was too skinny of course and immediately asked me if I wanted a rum ball. They were all lovely and very complimentary on how I looked but shocked. I suppose not too many people lose that amount of weight in a year successfully.

At this point a year into my journey, I was exercising daily either swimming or walking, and was just feeling amazing. What a different picture to the old me. I happily got out of bed and pulled on my runners every day. Something that I despised and really struggled with for so long is now joy in my life. Imagine if exercise became a joy for you? We all look wistfully at those people who are trim and fit – it can be you if you want to try.

> I was determined that I wasn't going to overeat this Christmas, and I didn't. While I enjoyed longer windows and family feasts, I was pickier in what I ate.

Appetite correction had kicked in so I simply couldn't eat the amounts I once did, despite loving all the food. I just had smaller portions of everything because I still wanted to experience all that Christmas fun, but I didn't have that bloated, too full feeling after every meal. I had really learned to keep things under control, even with my mother in laws divine cooking. That was such a good feeling and one I have never had over the Christmas period before.

I exercised in the morning and at least tried to get a 16 hour fast every day on holidays. I did it! It was the first Christmas in my life that I had put on no weight. In fact, I lost a little. That was a huge non-scale victory for me, and I really enjoyed myself too. I was so impressed with intermittent fasting and so proud of myself. I did a few 8 km walks around Sydney's inner harbour and I was doing that with ease. I distinctly remember the year before not been able to get halfway round on that walk fifty kilos (or 100 pounds) heavier.

So, 2018 my first full year living an intermittent fasting lifestyle. What a year, I had overcome my addictions to sugar and fast food, discovered intermittent fasting, and adopted it as a lifestyle. I lost 50 kg (110 pounds) in a year. My psoriasis had gone and so many benefits had come from transforming my health. I was so proud of myself and gave myself grace to really love myself more in 2018. That made all the difference.

> I finished the year a very happy man. I was super proud of myself that I had stuck it out for twelve months. I had never stuck with any weight loss plan or diet for so long with my weight in trying to get it down. I really started to see that this was just my lifestyle now, not a diet at all.

The longer I fasted the more I was enjoying it. I was a completely different man weight-wise by the end of that first twelve months on my journey. Still not quite there but not far away I felt amazing I couldn't believe this was possible in twelve months – well it is. You just need to commit and be consistent and the rewards of wellness will come. Imagine if you had pictures as I do on the cover of this book in twelve months' time.

I have watched Graeme transform over the past two years it has been incredible to witness. The wisdom he shares with others is testament to how passionate he is about sharing his journey in this book. As his employer, we are super proud of his dedication in finding his renewed health.

David M., Perth, Australia

CHAPTER 11

My Mate's Reactions

When I was morbidly obese no one who was around me ever said how concerned they were about my weight. The only time it was discussed was when I went to the doctor. Nobody asked me if I was sick or have some disease that was keeping me fat. Nobody said that they were worried about my health because of my weight – they just accepted my size. I had plenty of medical experts on obesity and weight issues dish out advice. I used to think it was funny that they were giving me advice when they were slim themselves and had no idea how hard it was to lose weight, exercise, or get your head around what was going on mentally as an overweight person.

I know people in my circle talked about my weight behind my back and I would hear that I was the butt of some jokes at a party. I was lucky for the most part people have been supportive and very complimentary about my weight loss. As we know, there is always that exception that annoying person or two that just cannot help themselves. The Neville know it all's who for some reason must comment on others' physical appearance. Usually, these people are far from perfect themselves, and probably jealous that you are succeeding at something. If you have been obese, you probably have some self-esteem issues that go with that. When you lose weight, your confidence soars, and for some people, it is hard to see you in that new light.

> **As I started losing weight initially, I thought I wasn't really losing much because no one commented, even when the scales were going downwards quickly.**

It wasn't really till a few months in, people were saying, "wow, you look good dude" and "hey, what happened to that skin condition you had? It's gone and your skin looks amazing". Then as I got down further and started looking like a normal healthy man, oh boy, I started getting it all and everyone had an opinion.

"We think you should stop now." "That's enough." "Do you have cancer?" "Are you unwell?" "Did you have a stomach stapling?" Yep, I had it all. I was 6ft 5 inches and 220 pounds so hardly starving and I looked fit and much younger than I looked before according to my wife.

I caught up with a few mates one day where we were watching Australia's famous horse race the Melbourne Cup in a pub. I was at the bar and a guy came in that I worked with for years in my twenties in Fremantle. I worked next to this guy every day for years in the eighties. I said, "g'day Steve, how are you going mate?" He looked at me like I was a weirdo and said, "sorry mate, do I know you?" I said, "yes mate, it's me, Graeme Currie." He nearly fell over and shouted, "WTF no way!" He said, "mate you look amazing and half the age, well done that's so awesome" and off he went.

Then my other mates I was with told me that they were going to have an intervention about my weight loss. "You have gone too far, and what's with these groovy clothes that you are wearing? You aren't a fashion model!" I laughed and got a guy to take a photo of the four of us. I showed them the photo and said, "we are all the same age. Who looks the healthiest, and the best dressed by the way?" End of the intervention, back to the beers, case closed. The funny thing was, two of those guys rang me later and said, "you do look good, we were just messing with you". That is what good mates do.

> If someone is not on your page maybe they are not on your journey to the new you. I got my mates on the intermittent fasting train now also and they are doing well – that's what mates do – support each other.

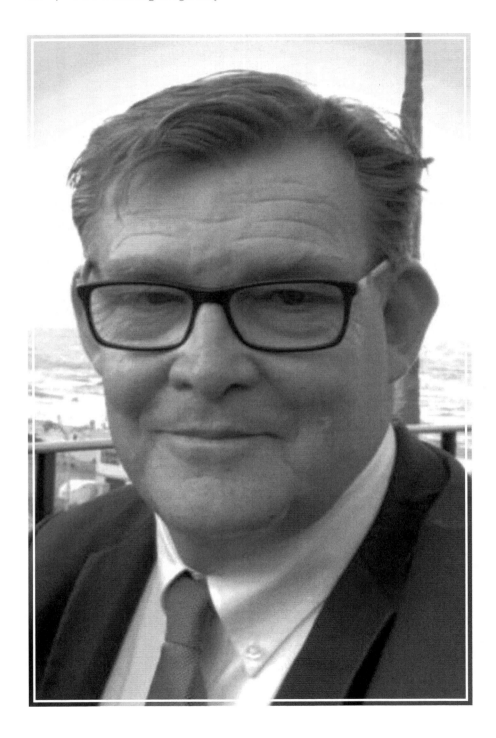

CHAPTER 12

Support from Family and Friends

I am lucky I have had great support from my wife and kids and workmates, and they are super proud of me. In a way, I feel weird when people say what a great achievement I did to lose all this weight. I did lose all the weight, but it was also me who made myself so obese and unhealthy in the first place. Support is important and my wife is so great. I have had my hangry days and I have had my "I am sick of this day" too. I have also had days where I was believing in my own success days a bit much and bombarded people in my circle about it after I enjoyed some success.

Initially, in the early stages, I didn't really share what I was doing with anyone outside the Facebook groups, except my wife. I was so motivated, and I thought I would just let my results do the talking. For most of my life with weight loss attempts it had been a lot of talking and not very good results. I just decided you know what? This time I am going to just keep this to a small group of people. I did have that fear of failure and looking foolish in the beginning because it was new, and I had no idea if it was going to work or had any clue it was about to change my whole life.

As time went by, more people were finding out what I was doing. My results were starting to be obvious as I dropped more weight. Of course, what happened then along came the naysayers. The predictors of my imminent failure with fasting, which some saw as a ridiculous and dangerous way to lose weight. I soon learned I had to stick with this for me and me alone. I didn't care what people thought. I didn't need to tell anyone if they were not happy to listen and I didn't need people to be a cheerleader or a critic. My mindset was I was my own biggest cheerleader and I was becoming more convinced that intermittent fasting was now part of my life permanently. My stock standard answer in those early days as well, you know, no one has ever died from not having lunch or breakfast.

It was so different, like finding a treasure map and having the keys to the treasure box. When I started to return to that goodness that was always there, experience increased health and wellness and the weight fell off me, I found out that fasting was totally amazing. I was getting some good early success and my confidence about it working started to grow.

I started to share more in the groups that I was in on Facebook. I started to feel comfortable enough to share more of my story and post before and after pictures to help motivate others.

It felt great and people were thanking me and asking for guidance, it was very humbling.

> ## Going forward, all I want to do is share this wonderful lifestyle with people.

This book is part of that, and I hope my podcast The Fasting Highway and my online beginners course for intermittent fasting can also help and motivate people. Pay it forward, get in the groups, post your pictures, and help motivate others. It is super rewarding.

The thing is, you can't let anyone take you down or belittle you. I did this primarily for me. It's a very personal journey and you don't need anyone to run you down for getting healthy. The rewards come for you in having a healthy body and that's all we need.

This is where that mindset, we talked about kicks in, and you can choose to let it rattle you or you can choose to let it galvanize you. I chose the latter, and I felt like I just needed to lead by example, and if people wanted me to share I would. I said to my wife when I get to goal and keep this weight off for six to nine months and I am totally in control of my weight I am going to help others. It has been a bit longer than that now so here I am. It was a big thing for me to see how I could maintain my weight with this lifestyle. I have done that now for over 15 months rather effortlessly I am hugely proud I have done that.

Sharing about something that you are doing personally just for yourself is one of those skills I have found that some people find difficult, for fear of not been accepted or ridiculed. As overweight people, so much of what we do is hidden, and the last thing we want or feel like doing is discussing something personal. They find it hard to talk about themselves and what journey they are on. If you start to lose weight as I did, you will soon find that people will ask you over and over about how you achieved what you have and why you look so good. Be prepared for amazement!

> I hope you do start sharing with others how great intermittent fasting is and how you love it. As you find that feeling of wellness on your own journey you will want to tell others.

We all probably have said to family and friends in the past, "hey I am on this new diet I lost ten pounds in three weeks". Then get the inevitable I told you that wouldn't work on that crazy that new diet of yours when it fails.

So maybe in the initial stages, just do what you are doing and keep it low key. If someone asked me about why I wasn't eating even at the start, I would just be honest and say what I was doing. I was just a bit cautious to share voluntarily at the start of my journey. I guess I was not sure how it was going to work for me and didn't want to have another failure. Now I want to shout from the rooftops about fasting and how great it is. I know that solution can help them, and it can be frustrating.

Its sometimes like keeping a secret and not sharing it with those obese persons that could really use some help. Then there is that fine line to you don't want to offend someone or upset them. I know how I felt when I was walking down the street when a guy shoved a pamphlet in my hand about a weight loss program. I asked him why he did that, and he bluntly said, because your fat and that may help you. Not quite the right approach and it made me feel so awful. I am mindful of hurting people's feelings.

First and foremost, this journey must be about you as we are all different. You need to find that niche, your own sweet spot the window that suits you the food types your body enjoys for you. So much about intermittent fasting is getting in touch with who you are.

> **We spend a lot of time concentrating on other parts of our life, and during a fast, you have a lot of time to think (because you are not eating or preparing food all day) about love, family, and personal self-development.**

As our thoughts move away from constantly been about food and agonizing overweight issues, it opens a whole new path to mindful thinking and developing new skill sets. So, don't be afraid to share without fear when you are ready you will have a lot to be proud of. I really look forward to seeing you share your story one day.

I have known Graeme for over 30 years he has always been an obese man. Watching his transformation unfold has been truly remarkable a triumph of the human spirit. The fact he has kept the weight of is inspirational.

Seth B, Perth, Australia

CHAPTER 13

The NSV
Non-Scale Victories of
Intermittent Fasting

For me personally, the most interesting part of my intermittent fasting journey was the much sought after NSV-non scale victories. These are the victories and positive things that happen on your weight loss journey that is not related to the scales. There are so many other benefits to fasting that happen along the way. What happens to your body when you start intermittent fasting will be different for everyone, but I will just give a summation of the main ones that happened for me.

Truly, apart from the weight loss these NSVS just blew my mind. If these are not a great motivator to take up fasting, I don't know what is. Once I reached my goal weight, the major health benefits were the reason I decided to continue my fasting protocol. I just felt so well and felt my body would continue to heal and regenerate and that has been the case.

For around 20 years I had unsightly psoriasis on my knuckles, elbows, knees, and wrists. Psoriasis was something that really made me socially awkward at times. I was always so paranoid that people were looking at my hands. I rarely wore shorts in the summer and living in the sunniest capital city in the world, which gives you an idea of how bad it was for me. I also had it on my kneecaps and back of my knees. It was red and angry, and I was embarrassed about it.

I spent a lot of money on creams and potions and went to many specialist appointments. I remember vividly a top skin specialist in Perth telling me that I had psoriasis for life. He apologetically told me that I was never going to get rid of it. He wanted to prescribe me all these creams and asked if I wanted laser treatment at a huge cost. I was resigned to the fact I had psoriasis for life on his advice. I asked him if it was diet related, he told me that it was nothing to do with my diet -yeah right!

> **Three months into fasting, I noticed my psoriasis started to look much better and seemed to be healing. Six months into my fasting journey, my psoriasis had completely healed.**

It was gone, and my skin was clear and looked great. I was so overjoyed, and my first thought was that I needed to go back to that specialist and show him. I have had so many people say to me, "your skin is amazing now, how did you get rid of psoriasis?". I have no idea about the scientific explanation. I have no doubt that intermittent fasting has helped me heal in so many ways. It is truly incredible.

I'd love to go back to those specialists who all have photos of my psoriasis and get them to recommend intermittent fasting to see if it could help others. So, if you do have a skin condition like psoriasis give fasting a try and see if it can help you, I can only tell you it not only helped me, it cured me.

> **I am pretty sure that a large part of it was diet-related and once I got all the sugar and junk food out of my system my body started to heal.**

I also think that the clean fasting and that period of rest time for my organs not processing food also helped. It really was like a regeneration of my skin, which now looks the best it has for over 20 years. One of the reasons I do share my story is I know how liberating getting rid of psoriasis was for me.

I know that the tone of my skin has also changed as well. My face has tightened up and my skin looks so much clearer these days. I know that my outsides are starting to match up with my insides. When I initially lost a lot of weight, I did have some loose skin but that too has tightened up over time. My jawline has become visible and I am much less puffy in the face. It is amazing how our bodies will respond in such positive ways.

I had was a dramatic increase in my mental clarity after beginning fasting, my work improved, and my concentration levels increased. I really had found true inner peace within myself my thinking and vibrancy were just alive and sharp. I had some wild dreams so clear and almost a replay of my life at times. Very early, on I had very vivid flashbacks about my life. I could recall things that I had never been able to before. Names, faces, and dates times came back to me easily in astounding ways. I can now recite the roll call and remember every kids' name from my class when I was six – it really is extraordinary.

> **Everything has just seemed more orderly and calmer now that I have been fasting. I feel more in control of my life in so many ways. I used to be extremely forgetful and would often misplace my keys and absent-mindedness dogged me a lot.**

My mum died of Alzheimer's, and this was always a worry to me that I would follow in her footsteps. I know that the fogginess I used to feel has gone, and my days are focussed, and my short-term memory is improving daily. I just had that increased energy and the way I processed things was much sharper more decisive I just felt in control when fasted.

I drive a lot of long-distance trips for my work in organizing events for farmers in country areas. I really noticed when I fully fasted how much more alert, I was behind the wheel. When I was obese there was more than one occasion I had to pull over and have a power nap on the side of the road I used to get so tired on road trips before I lost weight. I remember eating so much on a road trip once I very nearly dozed off at the wheel. It was scary!

I had for many years suffered from very arthritic fingers in the mornings. I would struggle to open my fingers on my hands some days when I woke up and it was quite painful. That started improving it just started getting better, to the point it just went away. I put it down to clean fasting taking all these toxins out of my body. I am convinced at this point the healing powers of intermittent fasting are incredible and wonder why everyone isn't doing it. I went through probably a good twenty years with arthritic fingers. I had rheumatic fever when I was a teen and the stiff fingers were a resulting problem that I was glad to see the back of. That was one of the best NSVS to be able to spring out of bed in the morning without the aches and pains.

I also had had a bad toenail fungus for so long, years really. I just accepted that it was there to stay forever as it would not budge. I had laser therapy on the fungus and used every potion known to man, but nothing worked. While that's been a bit slower to heal it's at least eighty percent better and looks to be clearing up. So many things just kept stacking up.

> **I just seem to be getting rejuvenated by fasting. I feel like my whole body was been overhauled inside and out.**

One of the strangest things of the lot was that I started noticing my eyesight improving. People thought I was crazy saying that, but it happened. My optometrist told me when I got tested that my vision has improved. He asked me what you have been doing? As I am a regular patient, and people usually remember me because of my size, he noticed that I had lost a lot of weight as well. I told him I had taken up intermittent fasting. He told me I wasn't the first person he had seen who had improved vision from a fasting lifestyle.

Not too many people in their fifties get that sort of report when they go and get their eyes tested.

> **The world seems sharper and the colours were more vivid. I really noticed when driving long distances my eyes were less strained.**

I now feel like a thirty-year-old man in a fifty-seven-year-old man's body, which is just an amazing feeling. I am more in tune with my body, probably for the first time in my life. I could just feel the wellness coming as the weight fell off me. I'm sure the main reason for that was the amount of weight I had lost. However, the other things happening in my body made the case for clean fasting to me undeniable.

Flying on a plane was the bane of my life as an obese person. it was just awful, and I had done a lot of flying around the world. I never suffered the humiliation of a seat belt extender or was made to buy two seats. I had seen that before with obese people at the airport and on planes. I got close to that a situation a few times and I was a master at hiding the fact that my belt was not done up.

Now when I fly, I feel normal and fit in just fine like everyone else. I used to get so anxious when I was traveling when obese. I would nearly throw up. It was a nightmare to travel with. Now I am chilled, and I don't feel like I'm about to be humiliated or discriminated against I just feel normal. I have to say feeling normal on an aircraft has been probably for me the best NSV of all. I look forward to flying on a plane now. It's that confidence thing again I will never feel out of place taking my seat again. I do a lot of flying and intend to do a lot of travel over the next twenty years and fasting has made that prospect so much less of a pain for me without being obese.

The other mind-blowing NSV was my dental situation. I don't have great teeth, to be honest, due to decades of addictive behaviour with sugar and fast food. I used to get bad gingivitis and when I brushed my teeth my gums would bleed and be inflamed swollen and sore. After about six months into intermittent fasting, I noticed there was no bleeding from my gums it stopped, and they were not inflamed or sore at all. Currently, my gums are a nice pink colour with no signs of gingivitis and my teeth look in much better shape.

> **My wife said my snoring had pretty much stopped as well. She said I was a chronic snorer when obese but never complained about it.**

I would often wake myself up, so it must have been pretty loud, and I am sure I probably had some form of sleep apnoea. Now I sleep well very peacefully and wake to feel refreshed and ready for the day ahead.

My wife said I hardly snore at all now and that must be so pleasant for her. Her own victory – getting a decent night's sleep!

> ## The thing that blew my mind about it was that intermittent fasting seemed to be curing things I had carried for decades in just six to twelve months. It made so much sense when I knew my body was getting that rest it needs to heal all these things.

There are so many non-scale victories that come from doing intermittent fasting and they still do for me even now. I really marvel at my own body and how it has responded to this way of life. I feel much more in tune with it and know that I am looking after it after years of neglect. That is a good feeling. Everyone who fasts reports something different that happens to them. I am sure you will have many of your own wonderful things happen on your own journey.

What intermittent fasting did for me is that it made all those painful memories of life as an obese man a thing of the past. Now that I am in what is considered by society in a normal weight range, strangers in public don't comment on my weight. They don't snigger and laugh say things like "wow, you're a big boy" or "man, you must eat a lot". I am just a normal average guy in the street now. It is so freeing not having those horrible comments. When you are obese you hear them nearly every time you go out of the house somewhere and it's awful.

I was at a doctor's surgery recently were on a referral note he had written, he described me as a tall slim male. Every doctor's report or any report I had been given in the past, always used the words obese or morbidly obese to describe me. I skipped out the surgery as happy as a clam. The laugh was that my BMI still said I was overweight, yet that doctor saw me as a slim man. He wasn't interested in BMI calculations; he just saw the visual. I felt normal at that moment. All I ever wanted to be was normal. I bounced out of that Doctors' surgery did a little fist pump and said, "I am normal" at the top of my voice. It felt good and it was a great feeling I have to say.

It would be remiss of me if I didn't discuss a very personal issue and that is my libido. All I can say is that I have always had a great libido even when obese. intermittent fasting has supercharged it! I can't imagine what it is like for my wife being with a man who has lost 60 kg (132 Pounds) but she is happy and tells me how handsome I am now that I am so much more confident. I think it's also part of the increase in my general energy and vibrancy. I feel like I have the libido of a man in his twenties again and it's been great. Just my overall men's health and wellness have improved so much. I feel very alive and very much like a very proud man.

> **Intermittent fasting and losing weight just gave me a huge boost of confidence in myself. I found my swagger, not in an egotistical way just the way I carried myself.**

For years I would sit with my arms folded as if trying to hide my girth. I would stoop over when I walked, and rarely looked people in the eye. I always felt inferior. Once I dropped the weight, that all changed. I looked people in the eye, I walked tall and straight and I now entered a room with confidence. It just was so freeing that all of that came about as I lost the weight.

To be honest I felt like the real me had been hidden in an obese body for years. In an overweight body, I lost that feeling of not been worthy somehow and certainly did not believe in myself. Once you conquer the mountain of getting rid of obesity, nothing will stop you. Being able to speak more confidently at events in my job was a huge bonus. I truly think that people do not think you are as intelligent when you are over-weight. They wonder about your discipline and your self-control, and I am sure this is reflected in how they look at you from a work perspective. I always felt self-conscious about my weight, like people were looking at me. It was very noticeable that the longer I did intermittent fasting, the more my self-confidence skyrocketed. Sounds quite good, doesn't it?

> **When obese, I had a phobia about been in public places. I was always anxious in big crowds or crowded shopping centres.**

I hated going to concerts and always felt like I was blocking someone's view and ruining their night. I just always felt people were looking at me. It would get to the stage I would often have panic attacks and just leave wherever I was. After a few months of fasting, I had a real sense of calm, and I wasn't getting anxious all that much. I stopped having panic attacks and I was just a much a more chilled person. I didn't have that fear of being in public and ridiculed about my obesity. My whole mindset had flipped around, and I was becoming happy with who I am, and my confidence grew as a result.

CHAPTER 14

Intermittent Fasting Downsides

When I first started fasting in the beginning, I probably was a bit of a hermit, stayed home a lot, and avoided invites to parties, work functions, and meeting friends for breakfast. I really didn't know how to deal with that situation at the start. I guess social isolation was a bit of a downside for me until I learned to handle those events and how it was going to fit in with my new lifestyle.

I guess I lost a bit of my desire to party go to the pub with mates and the invites soon dry up when they find out you are aren't the beer-loving guy anymore. I would say I lost a few people along the way that I thought were good friends but turns out they were not friends at all, more drinking buddies. My true mates just don't care if I drink water or whatever – they are just happy that I'm happy. As I got used to fasting, I realized that I could change my window if I had a social occasion that I wanted to attend. It was easy, I changed for that day then changed back the next day and got back on my 23-1 wagon. It worked and I was happy to be back with friends socialising again.

I soon learned how to deal with telling people about intermittent fasting. I had to – they could see that I had lost spectacular amounts of weight and wanted to know how I did it. People who knew me would look so amazed and immediately the conversation would be around how the hell I had lost so much weight. I was not used to talking about what I was eating, and often had a chuckle to myself thinking what closet eater I used to be, and here I was going through my daily intakes with people.

> I think I found constipation the only real bad issue I had with intermittent fasting. This resolved itself after a few months and now I don't have any problems.

I did also have a bit of bad breath or the dreaded keto breath, which also calmed down after a while – I just brushed my teeth more! Just on that note, brushing your teeth it does not break your fast and everyone will thank you for it so go right ahead as much as you need to.

One thing I do notice now though is how much more I do feel the cold now. I suppose without the 60 kg (132 pounds) of extra insulation that I had on my body it's to be expected. I do know people say they feel the cold a lot more during a fast. On the flip side, the very hot summers we have here in Australia are much easier to cope with without being obese that has been great. If a polar bear lost 40 percent of their body weight they would probably shiver too!

The only food I really missed was fish and chips it was always a big favourite. I guess in the last two and a half years I've had fish and chips probably about five times tops, when on holidays or out at a restaurant. I used to have it once a week at least. The thing is, I know what all the foods I ate in excess taste and smell like. I know it sounds weird, but I don't really think much about what I am missing from my diet now. I really do love eating healthy foods and the tug of all that fast food just isn't there for me anymore. My tastes have definitely changed, and I really can notice if a food is high in fat or sugar now when I take a bit and I simply cannot eat it.

> **There were moments when I was trying to get to the goal that I looked at people out having breakfast in a café or lunch and I would feel like I was missing out and have a pang of why am I doing this? Then, I would get back in the zone and concentrate on my end game again.**

The good news is now I am maintaining, I do a TMAD (Two Meals a Day) 16-8 protocol on the weekends so I can now enjoy that café lifestyle. I just go later in the day and have brunch. Then maybe a light dinner or just a cheese board in the evenings. That is something that makes maintenance easier, knowing I can look forward to those weekends with friends and family. That is the sustainable part of living a permanent intermittent fasting lifestyle. During the week if I want breakfast type foods that I love then I will have breakfast (Brinner) in the evening window. That is the flexibility of fasting – it lets you choose what you want to eat.

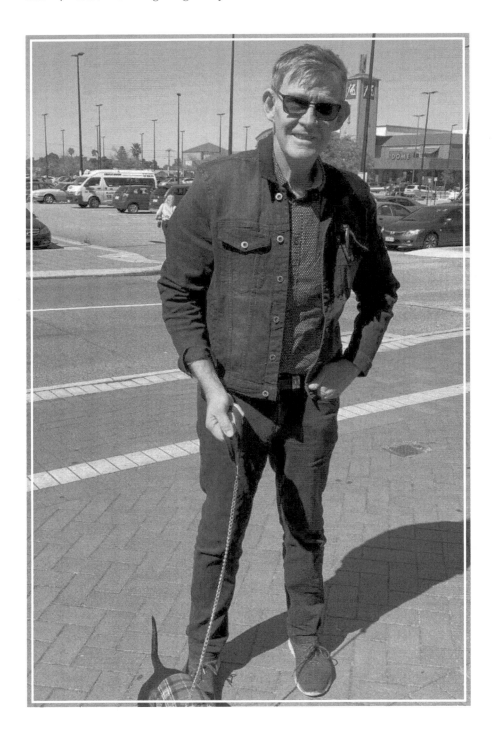

CHAPTER 15

To Weigh or Not to Weigh

Weighing is a hotly debated topic. Do you weigh every day do you weigh every month or not at all? Some people see no value in a number on a scale and prefer the way they feel or how their clothes fit. It really is something that is totally up to the individual and a very personal choice. You do you for you. Make a choice for you that makes you feel comfortable. You make the choice with the scales just like your window food choices any fasting protocol. Some people feel the scale plays mind games and find it tricky to cope with daily fluctuations.

Others love the science of weighing and the tracking of progress in numbers.

I am personally a big fan of weighing every day and do so. It's my accountability buddy and my truth machine that every day it tells me the reality of what my weight is. I also used the scales in my weight loss as a barometer to test out various foods. I got to find out the foods that my body reacted to weight wise – the trigger foods I call them. I just got to know what foods my body was hypersensitive to as well as drinks. I truly feel if I had scales that could have recorded my weight earlier in my life, I may never have got as obese as I was. We only had scales that went up to a certain amount I never knew for years what I weighed. The scales for me now have helped me develop a series of meals and food types that I know don't affect my weight much daily. It helped me identify the best foods to have in my window. A lot of the time foods I thought wow, I will gain eating that and I don't. Then there are the foods I thought yes, this won't make me gain, and they did.

> **So, my point is the scales became a great guide for me to ascertain which were the best foods to have in my window. You can gain in water weight and the scales will always fluctuate daily.**

That's why I weigh daily and average weekly works great for me. Don't let the scales define you and don't obsess over daily fluctuations and they do fluctuate. I can get out of bed weigh at 6 am have a big mug of tea and go back weigh again I will be up more than I was 20 minutes ago. Water in our bodies moves around a lot.

In my first year of fasting, I had quite a long stall for many weeks where my weight just did not move on the scale. I just trusted the process kept going and my body started to release the weight again. I did not ever have a continuous line downward. Some days I had a woosh, which is when you release water weight, and the scales move down more than usual. It can get frustrating when the scale doesn't move and you are doing all the right things.

CHAPTER 16

Exercise on my Journey

We have always been told you must exercise to lose weight – calories in calories out. To stay healthy, you must do some form of exercise each day. I agree with most of that to a point. When your obese, exercise is a real challenge, and it's for me it was just not fun. We all know we should do it, and I have probably bought every exercise gadget over the years to try and get going and get healthy.

The one thing that I did not mind doing was walking. I used to walk my kids to and from school each day. I really did not do much after they went to high school and when I was overweight, I did not exercise at all, apart from when they were in primary school and I did that short walk each day.

When I started on my journey, I was simply concentrating on getting the weight off. Exercise was not on the table at all. I wanted to get my food choices sorted and work out the window that worked for me to lose weight. I thought I would get into exercise once I lost the weight. I think this is a familiar idea that most morbidly obese people have. It is hard to go out in public and exercise when you know people will laugh at you.

My wife and I did start walking before the wedding to get in shape and we got pretty good, but it had dropped off after the wedding, and that is when I put the weight back on. When I started intermittent fasting, I was walking a few times a week but nothing serious – probably about 30 minutes. We live on a rural block, and there is always physical work to do. I would often be out of breath and have to stop frequently to have a rest from whatever I was doing. There was a lot of leaning on the shovel!

> **Coming into the summer of 2018/2019, I had lost close to 50kg or 100 pounds in less than a year. I started ramping up the walking out and added in other exercises.**

I just simply felt better with less weight, started to think that I could actually do it, and looked forward to it. I started to walk the trails around our suburb, which are so beautiful. I started walking longer distances to I got up to an hour a day about 6 km on the bush tracks around our property I started to absolutely love it. I would put on an hour podcast and off I would go. I listened to the intermittent fasting stories podcasts for motivation.

Never in a million years at that stage did I think I would be on there as a guest. I was feeling fantastic and as I started exercising more. It was a weird thing that had never happened to me before. The more I did it, the more I lost weight the more I wanted to do it. I discovered a new love for it without the burden of the weight it was enjoyable it was fun. Exercise became addictive for me I loved it so did my body I was feeling awesome. I bought a rowing machine and used that a bit as well as the walking I could feel myself daily getting stronger and fitter.

Looking back, I'm glad I did not punish myself with exercise when I was very obese. It was so freeing to exercise after several months of clean fasting. I had lost quite an amazing amount of weight off my body. It felt good I often wonder if I tried to exercise a lot when I first started fasting if my journey would have been as successful. When I had tried to exercise when I was heavy, I always ended up giving up. It was just too hard. I think deciding to get my food issues in check first, and then ramp up the exercise was the answer for me. The more weight I lost the more I felt like exercising. It was great.

> **Walking is an easy thing to do, but it is very hard to start. Give yourself little goals and you will improve slowly. You don't have to start with hours and hours. Just a walk around the block will do for starters.**

Work up from there. Be kind to yourself if you haven't done anything for some time. A buddy to get you out of bed is good – your partner or a friend.

Someone who will be on your doorstep and has agreed to do it with you that will kick your butt if you are not up and ready. Get your walking gear out the night before so you can put it on in a zombie state in the morning and get out the door. A bit of planning makes it easier, and you are more likely to do it. At the beginning of the week, think about which days you can walk, and which days may be off the table because of family commitments. Put it in the diary and make those days you can walk non – negotiable.

> **One day I was out walking on our bush tracks and feeling amazing. You know the scene in Forest Gump where his callipers break off and he starts running? Well, I had a similar sort of moment. I just burst out into a jog I couldn't believe how good I felt. I kept running and it felt so good that I could actually run.**

It was a very emotional moment on my journey I was like other people that could run and feel great. I could run! I can run! As tears ran down my face as I, Graeme Currie was running. That was an amazing feeling. I was doing something a lot of people take granted every day for that one moment. I can't tell you how great that was. I just felt like I was going to be able to do a lot of things I couldn't do when obese.

It is amazing how you get these turning points on your journey and for me, that really was one. I just got goose bumps writing that! I can run. Wow, it still catches me that one.

I started to mix up walking and jogging. I would run for two minutes, then walk a minute, then run two minutes. I was trying to learn how to run longer and get fitter. I am aiming to do a fun run in the future sometime when COVID allows us all to run together again.

Learning to Swim

I was always a terrible swimmer I never had any lessons in my life. Yet I had lived near the ocean for a big part of my early life. I have always loved the ocean and the water, it's a special place for me and has always been my happy place. I just could not swim to save my life and the more obese I got the worse at swimming I was. Of course, when I went to the beach I was always covered and rarely ventured into the water if there was a crowd. I was determined to learn to swim at the ripe old age of 56. It was going to happen.

I knew that they had adult swimming lessons at our local pool. My wife encouraged me, and off we went to the pool. The instructor, a very nice lady said ok, show me what you've got and where are you up to, so I know what we are working with. I felt like everyone at the pool was watching me on that day and felt pretty silly.

> **I couldn't even swim half the length of the pool. It was so embarrassing, and I was looking for somewhere to hide and wanted to go home.**

My technique was awful I just could not do it. I persisted with the lessons and went each week diligently. The lady was lovely and kept saying how well I was going. Slowly, I was getting better. I remember the first time I swam one whole length of that fifty-meter pool. I don't think I have ever been so proud of myself and it was a real sense of achievement. My coach was happy and everyone at the pool smiled at me that day. They could see the struggle and where I had come from. I felt amazing.

I started going every morning for months every day at 6 am up and down following that black line as swimmers say. I was doing a few laps without stopping, then,6, 10, 15, 20, and then I smashed it one day and managed 34 laps of an Olympic size pool – 1700 meters. I couldn't believe it! Me, Graeme Currie high balling up and down this pool in full flight. Well, it felt full flight anyway.

I got to this in only a few months and was getting fitter by the day. It was a day, like all the others and I was I fully fasted, and I just had this amazing energy burst powering me through the water.

> **It was one of the most incredible days on this journey that I have had and a truly emotional one for me.**

Swimming fully fasted and walking fully fasted is incredible, it feels so good. I've been walking jogging swimming and doing some rowing since then. I just love exercise as a fit, healthy man. It is my new addiction. Get me, heh? I never thought I would write that sentence describing how I feel about exercise but here I am. Imagine if this was you too!

I absolutely love swimming, and just going to the pool and taking my shirt off with no one batting an eyelid is great. When I was obese, I would never take my shirt off at the beach. I really think swimming has helped me tone up a fair bit also. I felt so much more confident with my body being seen in public and I felt like I belonged. The other seasoned swimmers always chatted to me encouraged me and re-marked how much I improved which felt good. It is great when people recognize the struggle and pain you go through when you are learning something new and encourage you along the way.

> I looked at these people and a lot of them were in their 50s and 60s and super fit. They are great examples of living clean healthy lives and taking care of their body. I was now one of them.

I heard Graeme on the intermittent fasting Stories podcast with Gin Stephens. He has one of the most inspiring weight loss journeys I have ever been witness to. It has helped me retake my own health by following his example.

Pat B., Western Australia

CHAPTER 17

The Doctors' Visits

After the first six months of intermittent fasting, I decided I needed a full set of blood results, so I went to see my local doctor. I walked in, she looked shocked and said, "you look great. You have lost so much weight Graeme; how did you do this"? I told her all about my journey and finding intermittent fasting. She was really into it and started taking notes. Then I went back a few days later and I got the results all blood tests were perfect, and my cholesterol and my blood pressure were spot on. My doctor said they looked like they belonged to someone much younger and fitter. She said, "your blood pressure is amazing for a man of your age."

She then told me she had passed on the name of Gin Stephens's book, Delay Don't Deny to some girls in the surgery who needed to lose weight. Now, whenever I need to go see her for checks she always is keen to know how the intermittent fasting is going.

It is amazing to see doctors so passionate about fasting and the evidence for intermittent fasting with obesity is undeniable. Credible medical papers like the one published in The New England Journal of Medicine, December 2019 have really helped convince some doctors what I think about the science of fasting. We, as patients can convince them by getting results and showing them that it works.

My wife fell ill with blood clots she developed on a long-haul flight coming back from the UK to Australia. Thankfully, she is ok and over several months was treated by a specialist at the hospital. Every time we went there for my wife's check-up the doctor would look at me and say you continue to lose weight and look great. I told her about intermittent fasting. On our next visit, she told us her whole family had taken up fasting. She was so interested in it and keen to learn more about it.

> **I guess there is no money in intermittent fasting. Imagine as an obese person if you were given a script with a fast, feast, repeat on it, and come back in a year written on it.**

Hopefully, that's happening more and more as fasting becomes an unstoppable juggernaut in our global community. I met a few doctors who sing the praises of fasting or who are interested in learning more about it. We all know fasting is becoming more mainstream out there and a lot of doctors are well and truly getting behind it in the frontline fight against the global obesity epidemic.

CHAPTER 18

Reversing Aging and Going on Vacations

Often when you see people who have released a massive amount of weight, they look drawn, wrinkly, and not all that healthy. I get told all the time I look fifteen to twenty years younger. People question when I post my before and after pictures if that really is me as I look so much younger. I don't really notice it until I get around a bunch of guys my age. When I used to look in the mirror, I would see a very sad looking, fat, a bloated man who looked ill and full of inflammation. I looked like a guy who was in his seventies. Now I see a fit, healthy man with a great skin tone and a guy who looks much younger. I have no doubt intermittent fasting not only heals the body it also reverses the aging process in a magical way.

I don't think I ever have looked so radiant and full of good health. That might sound vain and egotistical but it's totally how I feel. Gone are the days where I'd be asked if I wanted pensioner prices for a train ticket or at the movies at the ticket office. When my children were quite young, I was walking down the street with them. A street hawker asked me if you and your grandchildren are interested in this. My eldest said, "he is our dad!" very indignantly. Stuff like that happened all the time because of how I looked, and I am sure that every obese or overweight person can relate to this.

How many obese people do you know who look much older than they are?

I feel that fasting has reversed the aging process for me, and this has been one of the main benefits. I feel so much more alive at fifty-seven than I did at thirty-seven and I don't look fifty-seven- well according to my wife I don't. Aches pains and crumbly looking skin completely gone can say hand on heart that at age fifty-seven I really do not feel that old, I feel rejuvenated.

The great thing about intermittent fasting is that age is not a barrier to take it up as a lifestyle. I am glad I found it in my fifties and would encourage anyone over twenty to consider taking it up. I just think by starting young if you do have weight issues or are obese taking owner-ship of that early in life is a great thing. Now knowing what life is like not as an obese person I would love to have a lot of years back I feel I wasted. I really wish I knew about fasting back in my twenties as it would have saved me a lot of heartaches.

Vacations when living an intermittent fasting Lifestyle

In October 2019, we had a dream trip to Japan to watch my beloved All Blacks play in the Rugby World Cup. Japan is such an amazing country with wonderful people who are just great. The food in Japan is the next level and is based around clean healthy eating. We were away for two weeks and it was the longest vacation I had since starting intermittent fasting. I was worried I would regain a lot of weight on the trip. This was a rugby trip with mates and our wives, and they were all party people and traditionally I led the charge to the party. My close friends on that trip had also taken up a fasting lifestyle after seeing my results. I decided that I was just going to enjoy my time and forget about fasting for a bit. I did try to get at least sixteen hours a day in and roll with it if I didn't.

I hadn't had much alcohol in the months leading up to the trip and knew there would be lots of alcohol consumed on the trip. So, I came home felt slightly heavier, but not that bad and all my clothes still felt good on me. I weighed in the next day after coming home, and to my surprise, I was only up 2 kg (4.4 pounds). I had eaten a lot drunk a lot and we had the best vacation ever in Japan. The thing that probably saved me from really stacking it on was that I had been walking a lot in Japan – it's that type of place. Tokyo is massive and the train stations are huge, and you can easily lose yourself in the miles of walkways and tunnels to get to your platform. I never would have been able to walk the distances I did and combat the many stairs with my old weight. Walking around all day was a breeze and I loved every minute of it. It was another NSV that had a double benefit.

> I could enjoy all the sights, walk around all day, and still have a beer at the end of the day watching rugby with my mates – winning at life!

When we got back, I went straight back to my fasting routine it took me a whole two days to shed the weight gained in Japan. I was so happy I knew most of that gain was water weight. Which usually comes from carbohydrates that we have. I finally had this weight thing figured out. I knew I could enjoy myself live life moments without fear. I had found in intermittent fasting a sustainable health plan that was sustainable for life. Enjoy vacations don't fret, just go have fun. Fasting is a flexible lifestyle, just go right back to what you were doing when you get home. Life is short- enjoy your vacation without fear.

> **Once you have all the fasting tools you will be fine and will happily plan holidays.**

CHAPTER 19

Pictures and Recording Your Journey Along the Way

Taking pictures of yourself or getting others to do it can be challenging for an overweight person. We all have those pictures you cringe at, and I am sure if I asked you to find ten photos taken of you where your whole body it clearly in view you would struggle. We are the masters or standing up the back, or strategically behind a child or a bag across us. Anything that will hide us in the photo. What I want you to do is take a photo from day one. Initially, you will not want to share these with anyone. They are just for you. Down the track that may be a whole different story, so maybe the full-frontal nude is not the way to go. It's important to document your progress in pictures from day one. Even if initially you may not lose a lot of weight on the scales, you will notice changes in pictures.

Luckily for me, I had a wife who took lots of photos of me and I had a lot of fat pictures from my work and travels. I took a few more when I started but it wasn't really until my daughter's 18th birthday party while I was in that detox period, when I saw a photo of myself and went wow, that's a big change, even when the weight loss numbers were not that huge.

> **As I went along, I took a lot of pictures. I used them as motivation. I used those pictures to convince my mind I was going to be a healthier me.**

I also post a lot of my pictures in the Facebook groups not because I want people to gush over them or like them, which is nice. I wanted to show others starting out that this works and that I was living proof that it did to share and encourage. So please, if you're not far into this journey take pictures and compare them as you go. You don't have to share them with anyone, just keep a record for yourself and get them out when you are having a tough day to help you along. Nothing motivates me more than looking back at my obese photos. It is great to also have documentation of your transformation. You will never look like an obese person or overweight person again in a photo and will not scoot up the back of a group when someone pulls out their phone to take a photo. I can't express how good that is having a photo in a group and not thinking you will be the fattest person in that photo.

CHAPTER 20

Am I There Yet? Year Two of My Intermittent Fasting Journey

When 2019 came around and I was 6ft 5 and 108 kg going into the new year. I looked like a fit and healthy guy. I felt amazing in myself, and I was feeling so vibrant in my new body. I then asked myself the question, am I there yet? Can I lose some more weight? Do I need to lose more weight? I still felt I could lose a bit more, and besides, my BMI said I was still obese. By the end of January 2019, I had lost a further 2 kg (4.4 pounds) which is still around the average fasting weight loss of .5kg (one pound) a week. It was slowing down, but still moving down on the scales, which was great. I knew I was pretty close to my set point, the weight that my body knew was just right, and where things would settle.

I increased my exercise through March and April 2019 with walking and swimming and by the end of the first four months of 2019 I had lost a total of 7 kg (15.4 pounds) and weighed 102 kg (224 pounds). I really was starting to enjoy exercise and felt amazing. What a change from the guy who would not even get off the couch. I was daring myself to dream that I could crack the 100 kg barrier, a weight I hadn't been in over 40 years! That dream came true on June 27, 2019, when I hit 99.99 kg 220 pounds. I had done it. In just under 18 months. I had lost a total of 57 kg 125 pounds or over 130 pounds of my 2017 high. I felt so proud of myself.

I became very emotional because never did I think in my wildest dreams would I ever get to under 100 Kgs 220 pounds! Ever! I did it and it felt amazing. I was lean, without looking skinny or scrawny. I just looked fit healthy and totally transformed. It was like I walked into a room and went out another door then came back in as another person. I looked so different. It was weird looking at myself. I felt the same on the inside but outside I was like a new man.

I don't blame people for not recognizing me. At times, I don't recognize myself. It takes a fair while to get used to that reflection in the shop window or bathroom mirror. Or that feeling when you touch your body.

It must be so bizarre for my wife from going to sleep with a man who weighed 157 kg to 99 Kg. She says to her it makes no difference what weight you are. She fell in love with me when I was big and loves me now, just less of me. People who care about you deep down, are happy for you when you lose weight. I know it was always a concern for my mum that as a young adult, I became obese. I wish my mum were around to see my journey to wellness she would have been so proud of me. I ended 2019 at 100kg 220 pounds I had successfully maintained for 6 months. I decided to commit to fasting for the rest of my life – it just works for me.

CHAPTER 21

Maintenance

In July 2019 I started my maintenance program at my goal weight of 100 kg (220 Pounds). I knew I had to change things up and get my mindset readjusted to now make this lifestyle sustainable for life. I had lost the weight, didn't need to lose anymore but needed to get my head around how I was going to live this life forever. I formed a plan to keep my weight at a sustainable level in a tight range of 2 kg (4.4 Pounds).

When you get toward your goal weight, start thinking about how you are going to maintain all your hard work, and get a plan that is sustainable. It is just as important as your initial plan in getting the weight off. A lot of people get to their goal weight and have no plan to maintain. The great thing about fasting is the flexibility of the lifestyle. I knew fasting was going to be part of my maintaining plan. Going back to three meals a day with snacks though, just was not an option.

In maintenance, I do an intermittent fasting protocol of 22-2 Monday to Friday. Then a 16-8 protocol TMAD (two meals a day) on the weekend. I don't have two meals in my eating window every weekend, it just depends on what I feel like or socially what is going on that weekend. Sometimes, I just eat until I feel full and stop, not needing a second meal later. It is the same principle as when I was losing weight. I just ate until I was full.

My appetite tells me when to stop. It is amazing that I can now actually get those signals, recognize them, and do something as a result that stops my eating. For so many years I had no off button whatsoever. Those signals were missing from my life. Some weekends it is TMAD some weekends it is not. The freedom of being able to have two meals a day on weekends and maintain my weight is great.

> **I am still always a squeaky clean fast every single day while maintaining and that is something that is not negotiable for me.**

I have always loved brunch on a weekend with family and friends I found not doing that for 18 months to my goal difficult, but I knew once I hit maintenance that those days would return. One of my joys in life is having a leisurely brunch, reading the paper, and socializing if friends.

I was on a mission to get this weight off and keep it off, but I did miss those weekend brunches. Yes, I could have moved my window around on the weekends to have brunch in the weight loss phase. I just felt 23-1 was working for me so I didn't want to deviate from that until too I got to my goal weight. You do need to be vigilant with your weight spikes when maintaining. They can add up quickly if left unchecked.

I try to keep a very close eye on my weight and adjust accordingly. That is why I advocate weighing daily and taking the weekly average. I usually go up a kilo or two on the weekends and then it goes down during the week. I don't panic, I know what is going on and how to maintain my weight within a range.

Maintaining is a different mindset to that which you have when you are losing weight. Have a good think about is what a good weight for you. Our bodies get to a set point where it's comfortable and that makes maintaining easier. Trying to conform to a set weight according to things like BMI can be a challenge. The numbers may not match up and you may find you are happy in your set point, look amazing but your BMI will put you in an overweight category. Don't stress too much about it. You will know when your body gets to its set point as it just feels so right.

Once you are comfortable with that set point number and your body seems to settle there, it's great. My set point was 100 kg (220) pounds and that seemed to be where I found it easy to keep in a range of 1-2 kg (2-4) pounds. I have successfully done that for over a year despite a few vacations and many days that are not as strict as I normally am. This is important as this way of life must be sustainable. Do not miss out on important things like celebrations, this is for life if you want to make it a way of living.

> **I now have the tools to keep my weight in check and enjoy a healthy weight living a healthy sustainable life.**

I am fully committed to intermittent fasting for the rest of my life. It is important to draw a line in the sand and don't go up back past that line. If you do creep up in weight above that line, take control. Use the tools that fasting gives you and apply the same principals you did to get weight off don't fall into the trap of complacency.

> **I very rarely think or worry that I am going to go back to being obese again in maintenance.**

I do however remain mindful and I think that is important as part of your overall maintaining plan and mindset. I still hop on the scales each morning and that keeps me in my range. If I have a big TMAD weekend and put on a kilo or two I don't panic and just get straight back to fasting again. This has helped me maintain my weight within range easily. Not letting it creep is the key for me.

CHAPTER 22

Loving Myself First and Why It Was So Important

People can be so cruel and judgemental about body image. In society, you are either too fat, too skinny, too tall, too short, or ugly or beautiful. I can't tell you how intermittent fasting has improved my mental health. I had very low self-esteem, a poor opinion of myself, and was always conscious of my appearance which played on my mind a lot. Obesity is so crushing to our mental health and the way we see ourselves. It becomes suffocating deep down most obese people struggle with mental health issues.

My whole self-esteem and my entire existence are so much better now that I have lost weight. Those feelings of shame embarrassment and the anguish about my weight have disappeared. I no longer care about what anyone thinks of my appearance. I don't feel inferior to anyone. I feel so free and liberated. I am loving life post obesity. Nobody cracks the fat jokes or the smart remarks about my weight now. To get up every day, look in the mirror, and like what you see is so unbelievable, after years and years of avoiding my reflection and being ashamed to look at it. Getting through my day now is a breeze with the renewed energy and my mental clarity is so great. You too will find out what life is like post obesity.

> **I truly believe that looking back I never loved myself first, and that problem led to my obesity. I loved sugar and fast food first and I loved my addictions more than me.**

Once I learned to love my body, my mind, and myself first, everything started to connect. I was able to connect my mind to my body to my mind. I was in tune. I was in sync. It was just a process of telling myself daily all the good things about myself.

I learned to be gentle on myself if I had a bad day and learned to cope with adversity better. No two days are ever the same some days you will be hungry, so hungry other days you will breeze through the day. Intermittent fasting really helps you find that love for yourself and the feeling of total freedom that comes from finding inner peace. It's loving the way you feel and moves through the day unencumbered without food weighing you down, or the day becoming a drag. It's the love you find for your body as nurture it more.

Start praising yourself internally more for the good things that you do daily and let your mind open to your heart and get into a beautiful vibe without the dark days of self-sabotage with food addiction. I know this will sound a little odd to the blokes reading this book because we rarely look in a mirror intently in the mornings. It's usually a quick brush of the teeth and maybe your hair if you still have any and off we go.

I don't think I really ever looked at myself intently in the mirror when I was overweight – I just got in and got out as quickly as I could. Just take a minute to really look and have a chat with yourself – just inside your head is ok if you don't want to sound like you are going crazy to the rest of your family. These little affirmations every day will really help you, and when you start to feel and see changes, you will love the person staring back at you and smile. I know I did after losing some weight and still do.

> **It's all about learning its ok to have an off day give yourself some grace and get right back to your routine the next day. There is no wagon or horse to fall off with fasting; there are just moments in time where you are on a path to finding autopilot wellness and internal healing.**

It's such a joy learning the art of being gentle on yourself. Don't get angry because you had a donut or a piece of cake. Don't wake up full of guilt. There is no guilt with fasting and it's the most guilt-free lifestyle I can think of. Just remember if you are doing three steps forward and one step back you are making progress. Just try to keep the constant thought of loving yourself first, and then you can work things through and it is much easier than being angry or so in a hurry to get results you forget how far you already have come just by starting your new fasting life. I know in the early days I struggled with this but as I went along, things did get easier and I started to really look at things in a different way.

Now that I have lost my weight, I have so much more self-esteem, confidence, and swagger than I ever did before. I now love myself for who I am, and I don't mean that in an egotistical way. I don't have the self-loathing, woe is me, look how disgusting I look anymore when I look in the mirror. It's more like, how you doin' with a wink when I look in the mirror.

> **It is fun seeing that reflection with a sense of pride – so much pride. It's ok to love yourself and its ok to be in tune and be happy with who you are.**

These are the things aside from the weight loss that comes from intermittent fasting. There are so many NSVS, and so many little moments that most people do not give a second thought to, yet those who have walked the road of obesity to good health find so uplifting and exhilarating.

The other thing that came from loving myself first, as I discovered the taste of food and how good it could make my body and mind feel. For decades food was always was just volume. I was now finding I could taste the goodness and flavours. I tasted my addictions for forty years, and now I can taste the goodness, smell the aroma, and savour the food in my window. When I started loving myself first, I was able to pour love into everything I did on this journey. Now I am mindful of my body's needs, and I look after my mental health by thinking positively about myself daily.

I no longer stoop when I walk, I strut! I no longer sit in the corner withdrawn, insecure and broken, with little or no self-confidence. I used to sit with my arms folded over myself to try and hide my big stomach and my psoriasis on my hands. I don't have to do that anymore, and it did take some unlearning to remember that I didn't need to have those postures to cover my body anymore.

> **I learned to love myself first and the way I looked. It is invigorating.The more weight I lost, the more confident I became, not in a cocky sense in a way where I was happier in my own skin.**

I felt so much better just doing simple things like going to the shops for milk. Now I put on nice clothes to do that. I wanted to look good. I liked what I saw in the mirror and it was a whole new world from that abhorrent image I saw before. Everyone is beautiful but it's how you see yourself when obese that so soul-destroying can be. Mindset! It's all about the mindset. Please love yourself first – there is a lot of great things to like about you that I am sure.

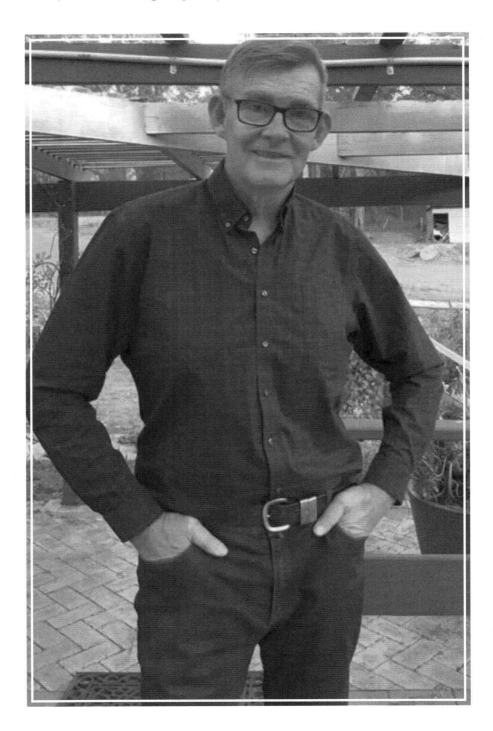

CHAPTER 23

Reflections and Goal Setting

I think it is very important that, when first starting intermittent fasting you have some sort of goal and to think about what you are going to do and how are you going to look when you get this weight off. What will my life look like if I manage to lose all this weight? What are the things, over the years that my weight has stopped me doing? What are some things that you would REALLY love to do but your weight stops you from participating in? Focus on that and let it be one of your goals, not just weight loss. Get a picture and stick it on the fridge of someone doing that activity. For me, it was so many the amusement park ride weight limits and riding a horse.

Riding horses is my wife's passion- she loves it. I would watch my wife ride in our arena or go out on a trail ride and wish I could do that. I was always too heavy for the horse and I am not a cruel guy. That day when I do ride is fast approaching, I can't wait. In New Zealand, there are so many exhilarating adventure things to do, and when I went home for a visit, I was always too heavy to do them. Now I'm not and I fully intend to try a lot of them on my next visit. My weight was always an issue trying to do things most people took for granted.

> I remember once going to enquire about a helicopter flight through the Grand Canyon from Las Vegas the lady said, "I am sorry sir you are way over our weight limit you cannot go on the flight". Now I can easily beat those weight limits and save myself the embarrassment and anguish.

I used to watch my beloved All Blacks play rugby and admire the big forwards of how to fit they looked. I often used to see the stats on the screen and wish I were the same height and weight as these guys. Well, that finally happened and it such a great feeling wearing my All Blacks jersey with great pride watching the games around the world. It makes me feel like a normal man, and it makes me feel like I belong in a normal world. You just need a few goals to work towards. Find anything that would be related to a lighter you that you want to do or participate in. Something that you can achieve and feel great about it.

> I really get annoyed now when I see a morbidly obese person get sniggered at or treated so badly. It makes me so angry to see people being so cruel.

I will never mistreat anyone because of their weight. I don't think people know what affect that can have on a person who may have serious mental health issues behind obesity. It's not fun being an obese person that is the butt of other people›s warped sense of humour who has no filter.

All I know is that now all those discriminations I found when obese are gone. They don't exist anymore, and I do get treated completely differently after my weight loss. The frustrating part is that I am the same person when I was 132 pounds heavier. Weight loss, when sustainable is great.

That's another reason I love intermittent fasting it helps keep the weight off as well as help losing the weight. It's a sustainable weight loss plan that can be implemented for life.

A transformation of the body and mind Graeme has inspired me to take up intermittent fasting. His passion to share with others is reflected in this book a must read.

Mike H., Western Australia

CHAPTER 24

The Intermittent Fasting Stories Podcast

I was stunned one day to receive a message from the Author of Delay Don't Deny Gin Stephens to say I had been selected to tell my story on her very popular podcast series www.intermittentfastingstories.com. I was to be Episode 23 my lucky number funny enough. She had sent me all the information as to how I hooked into the podcast I was so excited. I had never been featured on any platform where I was going to talk about something personal. The podcast goes out to thousands and thousands of people every week. As I got closer to recording the podcast, I became nervous and questioned myself and wondered if anyone would even be interested in my story.

I had beaten chronic issues with sugar and fast food then discovered intermittent fasting and had lost over 50 kg (110 pounds) inside a year so I thought that would be a good start. I was also eager to share and pass on some of the things I had found by living and intermittent fasting lifestyle to others.

So, the day came it was a Sunday evening here in Perth and I dialled in. I felt immense stage fright coming on. Then I heard Gin speak. In her lovely southern accent. I was in awe – this is Gin Stephens! This is the author of the book that was so inspirational in my journey. I was also so proud knowing I was the first Australian or Kiwi on the Podcast a real honour for me. A couple of other Kiwis have since been on the podcast.

> I had listened to the three previous guests who were like rock stars in the Facebook groups. I felt like I was walking onto a stage after Elvis, Springsteen, and Hendrix.

I was the guy following them, and the adoring crowd was all going to the chill-out tent because I was the lame follow up act. Right from the start of the interview Gins calming nature came through to me. Her soothing accent and kind nature really put me at ease.

I completed the interview and chatted with Gin while it downloaded which I actually really enjoyed, and the podcast was aired about a month later. It was truly an amazing thing to do. I was sitting there opening up to this lady across the other side of the world, an award-winning author about my personal struggles with addiction my weight.

A lot of people who listened to that podcast who had known me for many years were surprised at some of the struggles I had talked about, saying that they had no idea and that they felt bad for not reaching out and trying to help me. As a typical bloke, I was always very closed and guarded when it came to sharing personal, emotional aspects of my life. Very few people knew the real me, the food addicted me or the closet eating me.

I have to say if you ever get the chance to tell your story, do it. It is totally liberating to do so. The podcast was indeed my coming out in terms of telling some of my stories in a raw unfiltered way. I could not believe the response to my podcast and how far it reached I was totally blown away by the feedback in the groups and private messages I got and phone calls from people I knew.

People in the USA, Canada, Africa, UK, Europe were commenting on how they enjoyed it so much. I was getting calls from people I know who had listened to it and I was very humbled. The world is certainly getting smaller as we all relate our stories and connect around the globe.

A woman had said she was running in the mountains of Kenya listening to a download of the podcast. A guy said he listened on the way to work in New York on the train. It was so surreal people had taken the time to listen to my story. Here I was reaching out and resonating with people all over the world. It was wild my head was spinning. That's where I got my passion to share online my success and here in this book and on my podcast The Fasting Highway.

> I had a couple of farmers I know who had listened to the Podcast ring me and tell me that they wanted to try this intermittent fasting as they were truly inspired by my podcast.

Those two farmers have become part of a group that I help. They, in turn, help others. This was all from that podcast episode, that's the power of sharing.

> **Then I had a few friends take up fasting and I was so grateful to be given such an opportunity to share some of my story with others.**

I would strongly urge people who are starting out or looking for some motivation to listen to some amazingly motivational stories on Gins' podcast. This book and the start of my mentoring people all came about from that podcast. It just made me realize that my story was worth sharing. I also thought about how great it would be to help someone regain their health.

CHAPTER 25

2020 What a Year!

So here we are in 2020 wow what a crazy start to the year here in Australia. Out of control bush fires ravaged the eastern seaboard and a third of the country was burning. We saw heartbreaking news where people lost homes, lives and our native wildlife was destroyed in the millions. Then, after that, biblical type floods hit. Mother nature sure threw a few curve balls to start 2020 down under. Then just when you think it couldn't get any crazier, along comes COVID 19 that was spreading rapidly across the globe with devastating effects that are still in force today.

All our travel plans were put on hold and we were locked in our state unable to go anywhere. When the stay at home orders issued, I thought that would be a challenge with fasting a few meters from the fridge all day, instead of the office where it was easy. I really felt like I had to readjust my mindset again I always found fasting at the office easy as I just worked and didn't have the distractions of a fridge or cupboards full of food. We stocked up on food, as we didn't want to go to the supermarket as often out of fear of the virus. I managed OK, and just did my work from home and went for a short walk outside if I started to get tempted to break my fast and get on that slippery slope.

I felt it was the one thing I could control my fasting as the world spiralled out of control. I felt like intermittent fasting had improved my immune system so much, which is a great position to be in during these uncertain times. I hardly ever get sick these days and rarely do I get so much as a sniffle. We are lucky in Australia in that we live on an island that was easy to lock down our borders as the outbreak raged across the globe, and millions were infected.

Being in lockdown really tested my mindset.

I was living and working right beside the fridge all day. I could easily have dropped my bundle and eaten all day, worrying about COVID 19. I refused to do that. Historically, I would have stayed home in isolation and eaten up a storm. I refused to let a pandemic undo all the great work I had done with getting my weight down. I had made excuses all my life about my weight. I just was not going to let COVID 19 get in the way of staying the course with maintaining my weight.

I hope by the time you read this we have got through the effects of this awful virus and we can all start resuming our normal lives. I am proud to say I maintained well so far through 2020 and it is getting easier all the time as a lifestyle. It feels like it's just on autopilot wellness and I forget I am even fasting most days, as now it's just something I do. I still enjoy working out what I am having in my window I just don't have to think about it multi times a day. All the best for the rest of 2020 and may it come to an end quickly and we can all have a better year in 2021.

CHAPTER 26

The New You the Future

It takes a bit of getting used to the new you when you lose a lot of weight. I still have days where I catch a reflection of myself and go no way! That is not me.! it is not the same person in the reflections that I have seen for most of my life. I was taking a shower one day and while drying my hair, I turned and looked in the mirror. I shuddered with fright. I thought someone else was behind me and the reflection looking at me was not me. I truly didn't recognize this fit, healthy, much younger looking man in the mirror.

I tend to find myself looking in mirrors a lot these days because I like what I see. I took a lot of selfies of myself these last two years and my wife often comments and says, "really? Another selfie?" The thing is, I took those selfies to have documentation of my journey to wellness and pay it forward. I really hope that I can inspire people and show that a regular bloke can crack obesity that really brings you down. It almost feels like another person is in my body at times.

People do get used to the new you and accept it's how you are now they adjust. On the way down people closest to me commented a lot. now when I see them, they don't bat an eyelid as that is the way they see you now. It is quite bizarre at times going from a 160-kg (352pounds) man to a 100kg, (220-pound) man. I was cleaning our shed out and found an old pair of shorts in a bag that I used to wear at my highest weight. They were huge I could not believe how much smaller my clothes are now. I guess I will never forget what I was like as an obese man, but it is less and less these days. I had a guy at my office say to me recently I can't even remember what you looked like when you were fat mate.

> **Any scenario an obese person has faced I can relate to and talk about it. I never forget I was obese, and my compassion towards those people will never go away.**

That's why these online Facebook groups are so great because you are talking to people in the same position without the fear of rejection ridicule or not being heard. There is no one in there judging you or making you feel worse about yourself. If you are in a group and that is happening, I suggest you exit quick smart and get yourself another group to hang out with.

The acceptance I got from being a normal size guy to an obese one was so different. It really is a problem in our society the way obese people are shunned, ridiculed, and branded as somehow been lazy or stupid. It truly is eye-opening as to the discrimination obese people suffer. Wouldn't it be great if we were all just accepted for what we are? All I can say is life post obesity is worth the journey. It's a feeling I never want to lose, being at a healthy weight and loving life.

I felt like I had not only lost all this weight, I somehow had more intelligent because I was a normal-looking man now. People really treat obese people like they are stupid and lazy, and after experiencing and living both sides of the spectrum it's so noticeable. I often describe myself as invisible now when I am out no one gives me a second look.

> When I was 360 pounds and tall as I was at 6ft 5 people used to stare kids used to get frightened I must have looked like a giant to them. The feeling of the invisible man is a feeling I like a lot.

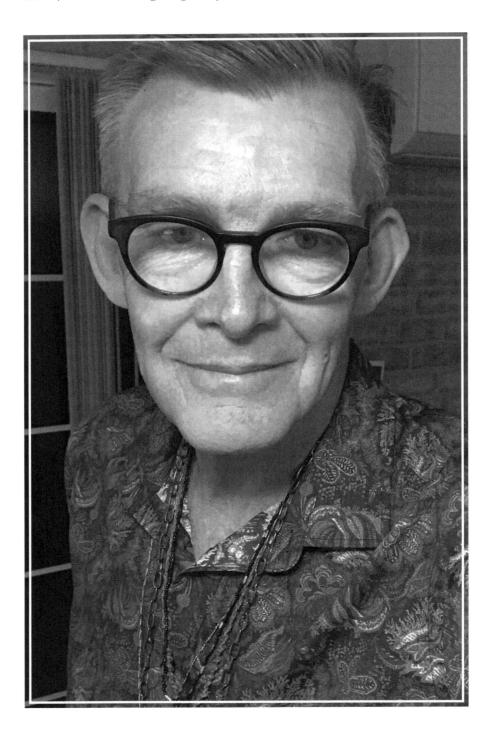

CHAPTER 27

Books Films and Key Influencers on my Journey

The following are some of the main influencers that I referenced throughout the book. All these listed below have had a profound impact on me and changed my thinking around food, sugar, and intermittent fasting. They changed how I looked at my obesity and gave me a lot of answers to questions I had for many years. I credit them with arming me with the knowledge to fight my obesity and retake my health and gain incredible wellness.

So, a huge thank you to all the authors below and I hope should you read watch or listen to my influencers that you gain the motivation to put all of these great ideas into practice. People pose the question, "can a book change your lives?" Well, I am living proof that a book did change my life. I hope they may help you as well as my own book you are reading now. I am not affiliated in any way or in the employment of anyone I recommend. I just found them useful on my journey and just a few of my regular resources I looked to.

From the outset, I said I didn't want to get bogged down in the science of intermittent fasting, as I am not a scientist. The reason is I did not want to do that is there is so much credible scientific information and research for you to find in one google search without me replicating it here.

Delay Don't Deny Living an Intermittent Fasting Lifestyle – Gin Stephens

Delay Don't Deny. Living an intermittent fasting Lifestyle is the inspiring story of Gin Stephens a former schoolteacher from Augusta, Georgia who lost over 80 pounds living an intermittent fasting Lifestyle I really loved Gins book it is one of the easiest and totally relatable books for anyone who has battled obesity and weight issues. It really is a heartfelt story with a touch of science-backed up with key links and references without getting heavily into the science around fasting.

I credit Gin with being the person who not only changed my life but likely saved my life. The book can be found on Amazon along with a Kindle and Audible version. I find the kindle version great as its always on my phone to refer to if I want to re-read some of the chapters. Gins Facebook groups of the same name Delay Don't Deny and OMAD One meal a day Lifestyle is fantastic, and I fully endorse joining them. Gin now has another book out called Fast Feast Repeat a very comprehensive book on intermittent fasting.

It will sure to be a must-read as it is an update to the science around fasting and the research that has been done since her first book was published.

I still read the posts most days in the groups to help keep me motivated to this day even a year into maintenance. I just find interacting with people there is very inspiring. I like to think that I can also help newcomers with some insights with a few motivational type posts. So, if you choose any type of support then maybe have a look at some of Gins Facebook groups and see if it would suit.

> **Thank you, Gin, from the bottom of my heart. We are changing the world.**

That Sugar Film, Damon Gameau

Filmmaker Damon Gameau documents the effects of eating supposedly healthy foods that contain high amounts of sugar. This documentary film by a very impressive filmmaker from Australia really made me sit up and take notice of the amounts of sugar we are consuming in considered healthy foods. A normal fit healthy young man takes a journey to see what changing his healthy diet to a high sugar diet as he travels and documents the effects on his body the results and effects the sugar intake, he was having were simply mind-blowing and distressing.

That was a real wake up moment for me when I watched it and scared the life out of me thinking how much sugar I had been consuming. I think this is compelling viewing in my opinion for anyone with sugar issues. I will leave the rest of the story for Damon to tell and its quite a story to tell. It highlighted to me how deceptive our food labelling is also in general.

Know what is in your food the key takeaway message for me thank you Damon for making this eye- opening film. This film really rocked my socks off. What really resonated with me was the amount of sugar pictured in a bowl that was in some foods and soft drinks (sodas). Every time I looked at food from then on, I imagined it as an equivalent bowl of sugar – it sure did stop me in my tracks. I still do that today.

A Life Less Sugar by Amanda Tiffin

A person with sugar addictive behaviour wrote this book. I could not believe my eyes how much sugar was in various foods that were listed in the various tables in the book. I learned about food that I had no idea contained such high amounts of sugar and hidden sugars disguised as names I had never even heard of.

It is a great story to of a Mum from New Zealand who lost 20 kg 44 pounds simply by reducing her sugar content from around 30 teaspoons a day to 6 teaspoons a day. She did this after watching a documentary called is Sugar the new Fat by Nigel Lata, a Kiwi psychologist and author, who thought the whole sugar debate was overblown.

Amanda was so taken she decided to immediately curb her sugar intake and researched the subject more and wrote her best-selling book.

She worked with her good friend Leigh Brown and published a series of low sugar delicious recipes in the book. It also has tables with so many food groups of what sugar is in what foods with easy to understand teaspoon icons describing the amount of sugar in the food.

Amanda is pushing for food labelling laws to be changed to make the food industry put these teaspoon icons depicting what sugar is in what food good luck. I highly recommend this book to anyone struggling with sugar addiction. It really opened my eyes to my sugar addiction issues. This book was a massive help to me, as I learned more about sugar in food that I was eating. It also gave me the motivation to dramatically reduce my sugar intake.

Papers

The most recent piece of great research I got something from was the paper released by the New England Journal of Medicine Effects of intermittent fasting on Health Aging and Disease, released Dec 2019 by Rafael de Cabo, Ph.D., and Mark Mattson Ph.D. You can find the paper in the New England Journal of Medicine web page at www.nejm.org.

To be truthful, for me the real science happened in my own journey along the way. I experimented and learned by switching things up a whole lot more about my body and how it operates.

I think no matter how much science of something you read up on or watch, you know your body better than anyone and know what it reacts to, or at least you will find that out with a fasting lifestyle as you adapt to it.

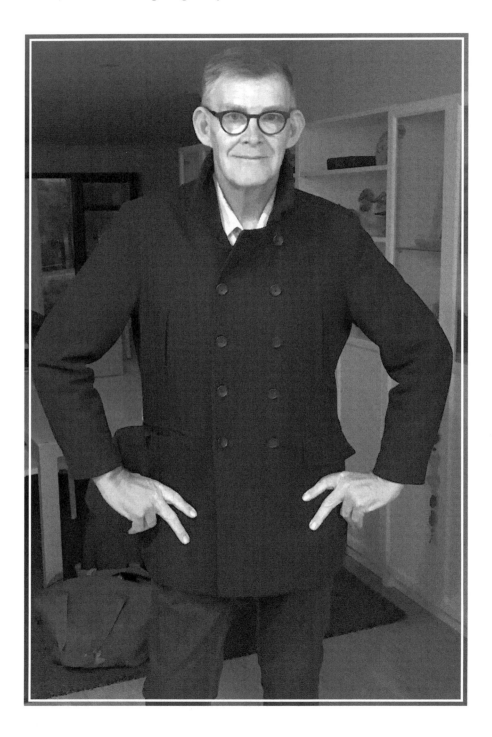

CHAPTER 28

Final Words of Motivation and Advice for You

I hope you enjoyed my story and journey on The Fasting Highway with, me and maybe you found some motivation from it to take your own health back. All I would say is if you stuck with me this far, give intermittent fasting a go. You have nothing to lose and everything to gain by finding autopilot wellness. I know you can do this for you. Stay plugged in to support and if you see me around give me a shout out in the groups.

intermittent fasting is designed to be a way of life. Free yourself from the burden of obesity. Address those food issues in your life holding you back. Start slowly learning as much as you can and ask lots of questions along the way. Choose a protocol that you are comfortably ok to start. Do not worry about what others are doing. This is for you and only you find what works best for you. Think about it do you want to change do you want to get your health back.

Look, being obese is hard, so is reversing that, but imagine if this worked for you, I know you want to live your best life and give yourself the best years you can. You deserve it, and your partners need you around so do your kids and workmates. The world needs you around. If I can convince one person to walk the journey I walked from morbid obesity to a happy, healthy state, I will be so thrilled. Take those measurements and tons of before pics before you start. Compare each month as you go note the changes. I suggest you weigh daily to take the weekly average. That is entirely up to you.

My advice is to give it a full 6-12 months then do a critical review. Tweak as you go play around with window lengths. I will leave the food choice up to you it is your eating window. Obviously, healthier choices in your eating window will likely yield better results.

> **At the end of the day, life is to be enjoyed so don't make yourself miserable. intermittent fasting is a lifestyle, not a diet – don't ever think of it as a diet.**

I know you can do this and I know that just by getting this book you want to do it. Dedicate the next year of your life to retaking your health back and live a life free from excess weight or addiction. Find a catalyst a reason to get you going. If it's this book you just read, great. If it is something in your life, for a loved one or a friend or just yourself, do it! Reach within find your inner strength to do this. I am so on your side.

Finally, a huge thank you to you from me for reading my story, about my journey. I hope if you are battling with weight issues that you try intermittent fasting. Honestly, it's the easiest thing I've ever done trying to lose weight. It's also the best thing I have ever done for my health and wellness.

> I wish you well on your own journey and truly hope to see you out there sharing your success to the world.

FASTING HIGHWAY PODCAST

If you are like me and listening to others stories of intermittent fasting helps you get inspired, I have a podcast called The Fasting Highway that you can tune into. I have guests that range from beginners to experienced intermittent fasters as well as leading authors, including Gin Stephens.

You can also visit my web page www.thefastinghighway.com. You can find details on all the podcasts and all things intermittent fasting including some before and after photos.

Email me at graeme@thefastinghighway.com if you would like some more information about private one on one mentoring to help you with your own journey along the fasting highway.

ACKNOWLEDGMENTS

I need to thank my beautiful wife Lou for her support right through my health transformation. I can't express enough how having a supportive partner has helped me get to this point. Lou really has helped me so much and been there on the days when I struggled. Or helped me get through the lows and enjoy the triumphs. Thank you my darling, I love you more and more every day. I could not have done this without you. This journey was so much easier with your understanding and beautiful kind supportive nature. Lou has been my absolute rock, my confidante.

Lou was someone to whinge to when the scales were not moving or someone to cheer me on when they did, I can't imagine what it was like for Lou seeing my transformation unfold. I know I was feral to live within the beginning of my journey. Having a loving and supportive partner is a game-changer as they really do play a huge part and, in my case, I had my biggest fan cheering me on every day. It is so much easier if you can get your partner on board and get the kind of support, I was lucky enough to have from my wife and family,

Made in the USA
Monee, IL
24 May 2022

96955776R00094